11-2-99

NUTRITION FOR THE CRITICALLY ILL

NUTRITION FOR THE CRITICALLY ILL

A Practical Handbook

Alexa Scott
Clinical Manager, Nutrition and Dietetic Services, University College, London Hospitals (NHS) Trust

Serena Skerratt
Clinical Nurse Specialist – CNS Nutrition, Formerly at University College, London Hospitals (NHS) Trust

Sheila Adam
Clinical Nurse Specialist – CNS Intensive Care, University College, London Hospitals (NHS) Trust

ARNOLD

A member of the Hodder Headline Group
LONDON • SYDNEY • AUCKLAND

First published in Great Britain in 1998 by
Arnold, a member of the Hodder Headline Group
338 Euston Road, London NW1 3BH

http://www.arnoldpublishers.com

British Library Cataloguing in Publication Data
A catalogue record for this book is available from the British Library

ISBN 0 340 69134 4

Commissioning Editor: Clare Parker
Production Editor: Wendy Rooke
Production Controller: Sarah Kett
Cover Design: Terry Griffiths

Composition by Photoprint, Torquay, Devon
Printed and bound in Great Britain by J W Arrowsmith Ltd, Bristol

Contents

Foreword

Nutrition in the critically ill has moved apace over the past few years. There is an ever-increasing realization of its importance in modulating the inflammatory response, protecting the gut, and stimulating healing and recovery. It now appears that not only the type of nutrition, but the quantity, route and timing of delivery, may impact either positively or negatively on outcome. It therefore behoves the health-care practitioner to be aware of its benefits but also the potential hazards and drawbacks. A major challenge also lies in achieving target volumes of enteral feed and in overcoming the difficulties presented by large gastric aspirates and diarrhoea.

All of these issues and more are dealt with in this excellent handbook written by a dietitian, a clinical nutrition nurse and an intensive care nurse. The unique combination of subjects covered in the book provides a broad perspective, which will be of use to any nurse, dietitian or doctor dealing with the critically ill patient. The authors emphasize a very practical, 'hands-on' approach, which makes the book ideal for bedside use.

Mervyn Singer
Consultant, Intensive Care
University College, London Hospitals (NHS) Trust
February 1998

List of abbreviations used

AA	Amino acid
AAA	Aromatic amino acid
ACTH	Adrenocorticotrophic hormone
ADP	Adenosine diphosphate
AIO	All in one
APACHE II/III	Acute Physiology and Chronic Health Evaluation (Versions II and III)
ARDS	Acute respiratory distress syndrome
ARF	Acute renal failure
AST	Aspartate transaminase
ATP	Adenosine triphosphate
BAPEN	British Association of Parenteral and Enteral Nutrition
BCAA	Branched-chain amino acids
BMR	Basal metabolic rate
CMV	Controlled mechanical ventilation
CNS	Central nervous system
COAD	Chronic obstructive airways disease
COP	Capillary osmotic pressure
CPAP	Continuous positive airway pressure
CRS	Catheter-related sepsis
CVP	Central venous pressure
CVT	Central venous thrombosis
CXR	Chest X-ray
DNA	Deoxyribonucleic acid
DVT	Deep venous thrombosis
ECF	Extracellular fluid
ECG	Electrocardiogram
EN	Enteral nutrition
$ETCO_2$	End-tidal carbon dioxide
FiO_2	Fractionated inspired oxygen (concentration of oxygen)
GALT	Gut-associated lymphoid tissue
GI	Gastrointestinal
GTN	Glyceryl trinitrate
IABP	Intra-aortic balloon pump
ICP	Intracranial pressure
ICU	Intensive-Care unit
IL-1	Interleukin-1

IL-6	Interleukin-6
IPPV	Intermittent positive pressure ventilation
I.V.	Intravenous
LCT	Long-chain triglyceride
LFT	Liver function test
MCT	Medium-chain triglyceride
MMV	Mandatory minute ventilation
MODS	Multiple organ dysfunction syndrome
PCO_2	Partial pressure of carbon dioxide
PO_2	Partial pressure of oxygen
PEG	Percutaneous endoscopic gastrostomy
PEM	Protein energy malnutrition
pH	Measure of concentration of hydrogen ions
PN	Parenteral nutrition
PPN	Peripheral parenteral nutrition
PUFA	Polyunsaturated fatty acids
PVC	Polyvinylchloride
PVT	Peripheral vein thrombophlebitis
RBC	Red blood cell
RES	Reticulo-endothelial system
RMR	Resting metabolic rate
RQ	Respiratory quotient
Sa,O_2	Arterial oxygen saturation
SAPS II	Simplified Acute Physiology Score
SCFA	Short-chain fatty acids
sIgA	Secretory immunoglobulin A
SIMV	Synchronized intermittent mandatory ventilation
SIRS	Systemic inflammatory response syndrome
TEE	Total energy expenditure
TISS	Therapeutic Intervention Scoring System
TV	Tidal volume (the volume of each breath)
TNF	Tumour necrosis factor
TRISS	Revised Trauma and Injury Severity Score
VCO_2	Carbon dioxide production
VO_2	Oxygen consumption
V/Q	Ventilation/perfusion
WBC	White blood cell

1

Introduction to intensive care

The aims of this chapter are:

- to define and describe the intensive-care and high-dependency environment;
- to define critical illness;
- to outline the support, drugs and equipment available in intensive care.

Defining intensive care

The Intensive Care Society (1990) describes intensive care as 'a service for patients with potentially recoverable conditions who can benefit from more detailed observation and treatment than is generally available in the standard wards and departments'.

The high-dependency unit can provide either step-down care for intensive-care patients, immediate postoperative care for complex or high-risk surgery, or a slightly more intensive level of support and monitoring than is available on the general ward.

The multidisciplinary team

The critically ill patient requires a vast range of skills and expertise to support the differing levels of organ dysfunction. Nursing and medical staff act as the orchestrators and co-ordinators of the patient's care and treatment, but input from a large number of other disciplines is essential. In the larger intensive-care unit (ICU), these experts will routinely include physiotherapists, dietitians and pharmacists, with a range of other professions, such as speech therapists and occupational therapists, consulted as required. The ward round is commonly the communication point for all members of the disciplinary team to discuss the patient, and active participation from all members is most likely to benefit the patient.

Illness severity scoring systems

These systems are designed to allow an objective assessment of the patient's relative severity of disease, and to enable comparison between different patient groups as well as different intensive care units. A large number of different systems is available, but those most commonly used are the Acute Physiology and Chronic Health Evaluation (APACHE II/III) (Knaus *et al.*, 1985) and the Simplified Acute Physiology Score (SAPS II) (Le Gall *et al.*, 1982). The APACHE II/III is more commonly used in the UK and the USA, and the SAPS II tends to be used more widely in Europe. Some scores for specific patient groups have been developed, such as the Revised Trauma and Injury Severity Score (TRISS) (Boyd *et al.*, 1987) and the Sepsis Score (Elebute and Stoner, 1983).

Other types of scoring systems have looked at the level of therapeutic interventions as a measure of workload, allowing unit activity and staffing to be assessed, e.g. the Therapeutic Intervention Scoring System (TISS) (Cullen *et al.*, 1974).

Commonly used equipment in the ICU

A brief description of common types of equipment and their function in the intensive-care unit is divided into types of organ support and monitoring.

Respiratory monitoring and support

Most patients in intensive care require some form of respiratory monitoring and support. This ranges from non-invasive pulse oximetry monitoring to the presence of an endotracheal tube and mechanical ventilatory support.

Pulse oximetry (Sa,O_2)

Continuous monitoring of the oxygen saturation of arterial blood (Sa,O_2) is possible using the detection of changes in the absorption of light associated with oxygenated and reduced haemoglobin. The ratio of oxygenated to reduced haemoglobin is calculated, and a level of oxygen saturation is displayed both as a waveform and numerically on the monitor.

End-tidal carbon dioxide monitoring ($ETCO_2$)

Peak end-expiration carbon dioxide levels can be measured and displayed either in a waveform or digitally. A sensor is placed between the endotracheal tube and the ventilator tubing, and a transducer measures the absorption of infra-red light by the carbon dioxide in the expired gas. This gives an indication of carbon dioxide levels in the blood, unless there is significant air trapping or ventilation/perfusion (V/Q) mismatch. It is useful for determining the correct placement of endotracheal tubes during intubation.

Arterial blood gas measurement

The variables measured in arterial blood gas sampling are PCO_2, PO_2 and pH.

Box 1.1 Normal values of arterial blood gases

- pH 7.35–7.45
- PCO_2 4.6–6.0 kPa
- PO_2 10.0–13.3 kPa

Derived parameters such as bicarbonate and base excess can also be calculated from these results.

Alterations in PCO_2 and pH have a metabolic as well as a respiratory origin.

Intra-arterial blood gas electrode

Continuous measurement of PO_2, PCO_2 and pH is possible using a thin probe, containing specialized electrodes, which is placed in an arterial cannula. This allows direct assessment of the effect of interventions and early recognition of problems.

Methods of respiratory support

The aims of respiratory support are:

1. to correct hypoxaemia and hypercapnia;
2. to assist mechanical failure (including an unprotected airway);
3. to decrease the associated workload:
   - work of breathing;
   - myocardial workload.

Nasal cannulae

These are short plastic disposable prongs that are placed in the nares, providing low levels of oxygen supplementation only.

Semi-rigid masks

This is a plastic face mask allowing delivery of low to medium levels of oxygen supplementation.

Venturi-type mask

This is a plastic face mask with a delivery nozzle incorporating the Venturi technique of gas mixing, allowing accurate delivery of medium to high levels of oxygen supplementation.

Humidified oxygen delivery

This is a nebulizer consisting of oxygen bubbled through sterile water with an accurate valve to adjust oxygen/air levels. This allows accurate humidified delivery of low to medium levels of oxygen.

Continuous positive airway pressure (CPAP)

This allows delivery of medium to high levels of oxygen with maintenance of a positive pressure during expiration, usually by high gas flow and a spring-loaded one-way pressure valve. This limits alveolar collapse during expiration and improves gas exchange.

Ventilators

The most common form of ventilator used in intensive care is the positive-pressure ventilator. This drives gas into the airway under a positive pressure, allowing movement of gas from the mouth to the

Table 1.1 Modes of ventilation

Mode	Description	Clinical use
Controlled mechanical ventilation (CMV)/ intermittent positive pressure ventilation (IPPV)	There are two types of CMV/ IPPV: type A – volume-controlled pre-set tidal volume and frequency of breaths are delivered; type B – pressure-controlled breaths are delivered to a pre-set pressure with tidal volume varying with lung compliance	Patient requires complete mechanical ventilatory support
Assist/control (triggered)	Pre-set tidal volume breaths are delivered in response to a patient attempting a spontaneous breath. A back-up delivers a pre-set rate of breaths if the patient does not achieve the required rate	Patient is able to initiate breaths, but requires ventilatory assistance to maintain oxygenation and CO_2 removal
Synchronized intermittent mandatory ventilation (SIMV)	Pre-set tidal volume breaths are delivered at a pre-set rate, but spontaneous breaths can be taken in between. Ventilator breaths are synchronized with the patient's spontaneous breaths	Patient is being weaned from ventilation, or there is a need for greater patient comfort/ reduction of sedation requirements
Pressure support (PSV) assist	Following triggering by the patient, a breath is delivered to a pre-set pressure level; the tidal volume delivered will thus depend on lung compliance	Patient is being weaned from ventilation, or there is a need for greater patient comfort/ reduction of sedation requirements
Mandatory minute ventilation (MMV)	A pre-set minute volume is ensured by either spontaneous or ventilator breaths. One major drawback is that this may be composed of low-volume, high-frequency breaths	Patient is being weaned from ventilation

alveoli, and inflation of the alveoli. Gas exchange of carbon dioxide and oxygen then takes place across the alveolar membrane. The positive pressure from the ventilator requires the patient to have a tube inserted into the trachea. This is known as an endotracheal tube, and it has an inflatable cuff to prevent leakage of the gas into the oesophagus and out around the tube. Different modes of ventilation are used in different circumstances (see Table 1.1).

Cardiovascular monitoring and support

Electrocardiogram (ECG)

Skin electrodes detect the electrical activity of the heart, which is displayed on an oscilloscope. Changes in heart rate and rhythm can immediately be identified and dealt with.

Arterial pressure monitoring

The patient's systemic blood pressure can be monitored continuously by placing a cannula into the artery and attaching it to a fluid-filled transducer. The transducer transmits changes in pressure as changes in electricity, which are picked up and displayed both as a waveform and digitally by the monitor.

Central venous pressure monitoring

Central vein pressures can be monitored via a central venous cannula using the same technique as that described above.

Pulmonary artery catheters

A catheter can be passed into the pulmonary artery from a central vein via the right atrium and ventricle. Pressure is then transduced to produce a waveform and digital read-out on the monitor. Pulmonary artery pressures give an indication of pressures on the left side of the heart which cannot be monitored directly. The pulmonary artery catheter incorporates a balloon near the tip, which can be inflated. When inflation occurs in a small pulmonary vessel, that vessel is occluded and pressure can be measured at the tip of the pulmonary catheter. This is without the influence of pressures from the right side of the heart. This pressure reflects the left ventricular pressure and diastolic pressure, and gives an indication of fluid volumes on the left side of the heart.

Cardiac output studies

Cardiac output is the volume of blood ejected by the ventricles over a period of 1 min, and it can be measured using a thermodilution technique from the pulmonary artery catheter. A known quantity of fluid at a known temperature (room temperature or below) is injected into the right atrium. Its dilution by the blood flow is calculated from serial changes in blood temperature measured in the pulmonary artery. Further calculations including stroke volume, systemic vascular resistance and pulmonary vascular resistance can be made.

Doppler ultrasound

Another technique for measuring cardiac output makes use of Doppler ultrasound. This measures blood flow using the change in frequency associated with reflection of the sound by moving blood corpuscles. The Doppler probe is placed in the oesophagus and positioned by the descending thoracic aorta. Blood flow through the aorta is measured and cardiac output calculated using a nomogram incorporating the patient's height, weight and age.

Pacing

When the normal pacemaker of the heart (the sino-atrial node) fails, or conduction of the signal through the heart becomes unreliable, a contraction can be stimulated by the passage of a small current of electrical energy delivered to the heart. In a temporary situation the current can be delivered externally, through a central vein, or through wires attached during cardiac surgery. Permanent pacing systems require an implantable generator.

Intra-aortic balloon pump (IABP)

The IABP is used to provide short-term support of the heart in cardiogenic shock and/or following cardiopulmonary bypass. A balloon attached to a catheter is inserted into the descending aorta. A pump shuttles helium under pressure through the catheter to inflate and deflate the balloon in time with the contraction and relaxation of the heart. The balloon inflates during relaxation and deflates with contraction.

Renal replacement therapy

Many critically ill patients require renal support, and those who develop renal failure will require renal replacement therapy.

A range of differing techniques has been designed to remove fluid and solutes that are normally excreted by the kidney. All of them, apart from peritoneal dialysis, require blood to be pumped extracorporeally and carry risks to both patient and staff as a result.

Box 1.2 Types of renal replacement therapy

- *Haemofiltration* (various types) – a convective process with mass movement of plasma, water and solutes across a highly permeable membrane
- *Haemodiafiltration* (various types) – the efficiency of haemofiltration can be improved by running dialysis solution on the opposite side of the membrane utilizing diffusion to increase solute removal
- *Intermittent haemodialysis* – high flow rates of blood are passed through a semi-permeable membrane with a dialysis solution on the opposite side increasing solute removal. Fluid is removed by ultrafiltration. The technique is faster than haemofiltration or diafiltration
- *Peritoneal dialysis* – the peritoneum is used as a membrane across which solutes pass into a dialysis fluid. Fluid is removed using an osmotic gradient provided by varying ranges of glucose concentration

---

Intracranial pressure (ICP) monitoring

Continuous monitoring of intracranial pressure allows early intervention to prevent high and potentially damaging pressures and evaluation of the effect of patient care on the ICP. The commonest technique involves the placement of a rigid bolt through a burr hole into the subdural space. This is connected to a fluid-filled system or a transducer allowing measurement of pressure.

Table 1.2 Drugs commonly used in the ICU

Type of drug	Examples of drug	Effect
Opioid analgesics	Morphine, papaveretum, pethidine, Fentanyl, Alfentanil, etc.	Analgesia, when patient is ventilated, may also be used for suppression of respiratory drive
Sedatives	Midazolam, propofol, diazepam, lorazepam	Sedation/anaesthesia
Muscle relaxants	Pancuronium, atracurium, vecuronium	Skeletal muscle relaxation to facilitate intubation and/or ventilation
Inotropes	Adrenaline, noradrenaline, dobutamine, dopexamine, dopamine	Increased contractility of the myocardium, thereby increasing cardiac output
Vasodilators	Sodium nitroprusside, glyceryl trinitrate, isosorbide trinitrate	Vasodilation of arteries and/or veins, thus reducing resistance to circulatory blood flow
Anti-arrhythmics	Adenosine, Amiodarone, digoxin, Verapamil, lignocaine, magnesium	Decreased excitation or conduction of fast or abnormal heart rhythms
Antifibrinolytics	Tranexamic acid, aprotinin	Prevent the lysis of clot formation
Thrombolytics	Streptokinase, tissue plasminogen activator, urokinase	Dissolve clots
Anticoagulants	Heparin, prostacyclin	Prevent clot formation
Bronchodilators	Salbutamol, aminophylline, ipratropium	Dilation of bronchioles in bronchospasm, asthma and chronic obstructive airways disease (COAD)

Table 1.3 Drugs affecting gastrointestinal function that are used in the critically ill

Drug type	Drug	Effect
Drugs affecting gastrointestinal perfusion	Adrenaline Noradrenaline	Affect predominantly α-receptors at high doses (adrenaline > 0.2 μg/kg/min and noradrenaline >4 μg/kg/min), with resultant splanchnic vasoconstriction
	Dopamine	Low doses (2–5 μg/kg/min) act on β_2 and DA_1 receptors, relaxing vascular smooth muscle. DA_1 effect may be protective even during α-receptor stimulation. High doses cause intense vasoconstriction via α-receptor stimulation.
	Dopexamine	Improves splanchnic and renal perfusion via β_2 and DA receptor stimulation
	Isoprenaline	Improves splanchnic and renal perfusion
	Digoxin	Constricts mesenteric vasculature
Drugs affecting gastrointestinal flora	Antibiotics, particularly broad-spectrum, e.g. cephalosporins and ampicillin	Disturbs the balance of commensal to pathogenic flora, allowing proliferation of pathogens
Drugs used in prevention of gastrointestinal bleeding	Vasopressin	Potent vasoconstrictor, reducing splanchnic blood flow and hepatoportal pressure
	Tranexamic acid	Antifibrinolytic
	Aprotinin	Antifibrinolytic
	Desmopressin	Causes release of plasma von Willebrand's factor and ethamsylate which stabilizes platelet adhesion
	Somatostatin/octeotide	Reduces gastric acid and pancreatic secretion, gastrointestinal blood flow, small intestine transit and nutrient absorption

Anti-diarrhoeal agents	Loperamide	Reduces gastrointestinal motility and secretions by interacting with opioid and cholinergic receptors
	Codeine Phosphate	Opioid action inhibiting non-adrenergic and non-cholinergic nerves and exciting cholinergic nerves, reducing peristalsis
	Lomotil (diphenoxylate and atropine)	Produces a similar effect to codeine phosphate
Prokinetic agents	Metaclopromide	Increases gastric emptying, duodenal/jejunal motility and gastro-oesophageal tone
	Cisapride	Promotes oesophageal, small intestinal and colonic motility, and increases gastric motility (more potent than metaclopromide)
	Erythromycin	Motilin-binding inhibitor with gastric prokinetic properties
Enteral feed/nutrition interaction	Phenytoin	Level of activity of phenytoin is reduced
Drugs reducing gastrointestinal motility	Opiates, e.g. morphine	Delayed gastric emptying, reduced biliary and pancreatic secretions, diminished propulsive contractions in small and large intestine
Drugs promoting osmotic diarrhoea	Sorbitol containing oral syrups, e.g. KCL syrup	Excess amounts can increase intraluminal osmolarity producing movement of fluid into the gut and causing diarrhoea
Laxative agents	Osmotic laxatives, e.g. lactulose, sorbitol	Lactulose is metabolized to lactate and other organic acids by colonic bacteria. These substances exert an osmotic effect and increase stool water
	Stimulant laxatives, e.g. senna, bisacodyl	These stimulate the myenteric plexus, inducing increased smooth muscle contraction

α-receptors, stimulation causes vasoconstriction of smooth muscle; β-receptors, stimulation causes increased heart rate and contractility; β_2-receptors, stimulation causes arteriolar vasodilation and bronchodilation; DA_1 receptors, stimulation causes vasodilation of splanchnic circulation, increasing renal blood flow.

Drugs commonly used in the ICU

These are summarized in Table 1.2. Drugs which affect gastro-intestinal function are listed in Table 1.3.

References

Boyd, C.R., Tolson, M.A. and Copes, W.S. 1987: Evaluating trauma care: the TRISS method. *Journal of Trauma* **27**, 370–78.

Cullen, D.J., Civetta, J.M., Briggs, B.A. and Ferrara, L.C. 1974: Therapeutic intervention scoring system: a method for quantitative comparison of patient care. *Critical Care Medicine* **2**, 57–60.

Elebute, E.A. and Stoner, H.B. 1983: The grading of sepsis. *British Journal of Surgery* **70**, 29–31.

Intensive Care Society 1990: *The intensive care service in the UK*. London: Intensive Care Society.

Knaus, W.A., Draper, E.A., Wagner, D.P. and Zimmerman, J.E. 1985: APACHE II: a severity of disease classification system. *Critical Care Medicine* **13**, 818–29.

Le Gall, J., Brun-Buisson, C., Trunet, P., Latournerie, J., Cantereau, S. and Rapin, M. 1982: Influence of age, previous health status, and severity of acute illness on outcome from intensive care. *Critical Care Medicine* **10**, 575–7.

Further reading

Adam, S.K. and Osborne, S. 1997: *Critical care nursing: science and practice*. Oxford: Oxford University Press.

2

The stress response and the role of nutrition in the critically ill patient

The aims of this chapter are:
- to provide an overview of normal metabolism;
- to describe the feed/fast cycle in humans and the hypermetabolic response to trauma/injury;
- to explain the role of nutrition and novel substrates in the critically ill patient, and the rationale for feeding.

An overview of normal metabolism

In the healthy individual normal cellular metabolism is dependent on:
- adequate oxygenation;
- substrate delivery and utilization (the substrates that provide energy for metabolism are carbohydrate, fat, and protein);
- excretion of metabolites and waste products.

When food is ingested, carbohydrate, fat and protein are oxidized to produce energy, carbon dioxide and water, and heat is generated as a by-product.

The energy released from this process is expressed in kilocalories (kcal), and can be converted to potential energy as adenosine triphosphate (ATP). This potential energy can be used as fuel for physical work. For example:

Expired via lungs

$$O_2 + \text{fuel source (e.g. } C_6H_{12}O_6) = 6\,CO_2 + 6\,H_2O + \text{energy}$$

Excreted

- Oxidation of 1 g of carbohydrate yields 3.75 kcal of energy.
- Oxidation of 1 g of fat yields 9 kcal of energy.
- Oxidation of 1 g of protein yields 4 kcal of energy.

Carbohydrate, fat (lipids) and protein are oxidized at different rates under different metabolic conditions. In addition, specific tissues show a preference for different substrates.

For example, the brain, renal medulla, lens of the eye and red blood cells have a specific requirement for glucose as a fuel. The location of the major metabolic pathways is shown in Fig. 2.1.

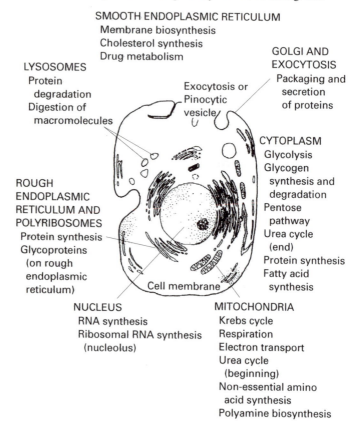

Fig. 2.1 Cellular location of major metabolic pathways. (Luker, M.C. (ed.) 1991: *Nutritional Biochemistry and metabolism with clinical applications*, 2nd edn. Amsterdam: Elsevier.)

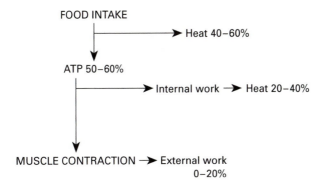

Fig. 2.2 Energy transfer in humans. (Adapted from Long, J.M. and Long, C.L. 1994: Fuel metabolism. In Zaloga, G.P. (ed.) *Nutrition in critical care.* Mosby: St Louis, 36.)

Energy requirements can only be sustained by the continuous provision of predominantly ATP plus other high-energy phosphate compounds, e.g. phosphocreatine in muscles, and adenosine diphosphate (ADP) – the energy currency of the cells. The reactions involved in energy transfer in humans are summarized in Fig. 2.2.

Energy requirements can be determined from an estimation of the metabolic rate, which is the rate at which energy is expended in various metabolic processes.

The *total energy expenditure* (TEE) is composed of the following;

- the basal metabolic rate (BMR), which accounts for 60 to 70 per cent of TEE (this is a standardized measurement);
- physical activity;
- thermogenesis, i.e. the energy expended over and above BMR and physical activity. This includes the effects of food intake, cold exposure, thermogenic agents and stress.

The term *basal metabolic rate* refers to energy expended by the individual in strictly controlled conditions over a 24-h period, and reflects the energy required to maintain essential body structure and functions, e.g. cell synthesis and regeneration.

In practice, the *resting metabolic rate* (RMR) is used to estimate requirements in the clinical setting, because even when resting the patient is rarely in basal conditions. The RMR accounts for 60 to 79 per cent of the total energy expenditure.

The *resting metabolic rate* is defined as the rate of energy expended by resting healthy individuals or ill subjects who are not in thermoneutral conditions. In addition, they may be pyrexial, on medication, and receiving nutritional support and/or other supportive treatments.

RMR is governed by the following factors, all of which are relevant to the ICU patient, with the exception of activity level:

- basal requirements;
- age, sex, weight and height;
- activity level (not generally applicable in critically ill patients);
- pain and anxiety;
- ambient temperature;
- diet-induced thermogenesis, i.e. energy produced during the oxidation and processing of foods consumed. This will also apply to patients receiving parenteral nutrition.

The most accurate ways of measuring energy expenditure are:

- by calorimetry;
- by the double-labelled radio-isotope water method, which is too expensive to be carried out routinely.

Indirect calorimetry is the measurement of energy expenditure from oxygen consumption and carbon dioxide production, and is only used for research purposes in the critically ill. It is inaccurate in patients requiring >60 per cent inspired oxygen or in those on continuous renal replacement therapy, due to carbon dioxide losses across the haemofilter.

Direct calorimetry measures the amount of heat produced by the individual, and is never used in practice because it is too restrictive

Table 2.1 Energy consumption in humans

Description/activity	Energy use
Normal adult female	1700–2000 kcal/day
Normal adult male	2400–2800 kcal/day
Bedridden patient	1300–1800 kcal/day
Critically ill patient	1700–2500 kcal/day
Sitting at rest	0.7–2.0 kcal/min
Walking	2.0–6.0 kcal/min
Sprinting	≥15 kcal/min

(Adapted from Halperin, M.L. and Rolleston, F.S. 1993: Energy fuels and stores. In *Clinical detection stories: A problem-based approach to clinical cases in energy and acid-base metabolism.* Portland Press: London and Chapel Hill, 4.)

to be utilized in the ICU setting. It is also expensive and requires a skilled operator.

In practice, formulae are used to predict BMR and requirements in the critically ill (see Chapter 3).

In trauma and sepsis, a measurement of resting energy expenditure approximates closely to total energy expenditure, as drugs used routinely in ICU, such as sedatives and paralysing agents, can reduce TEE (see Table 2.1).

Activities/interventions that can increase or decrease energy consumption in the critically ill patient include:

- rest;
- bathing;
- sleep;
- drug therapy, e.g. muscle relaxants;
- presence of visitors;
- physiotherapy;
- dressing changes;
- positioning for chest X-ray.

Weissman *et al.* (1984) measured eight basic ICU activities and found that the highest energy expenditure occurred during chest physiotherapy.

Prior to a consideration of the metabolic response to injury, it is important to appreciate the normal feed/fast cycle in the healthy individual.

Feed/fast cycle

Man is an intermittent feeder, and therefore the body has to adapt to both periods of surfeit after a meal (postprandial) and periods of fasting (e.g. overnight when asleep). There is therefore a requirement for surplus nutrients to be stored in a form that is readily available in times of fasting.

Postprandial period

Following a conventional meal, blood sugar levels rise and the hormone insulin is secreted to facilitate the transport of glucose into the cells and to decrease the elevated blood sugar level.

The effects of insulin are tissue specific, particularly affecting skeletal muscle and adipose tissue. In muscle, insulin accelerates the transport of glucose into the cells, enhances the synthesis of glycogen (the storage form of glucose) and increases the synthesis of muscle protein. The net effect is that glucose is provided as energy for contraction of muscles, while glycogen is stored as a readily accessible fuel for any future deficits.

In adipose tissue, insulin promotes fat production and storage in adipocytes, and simultaneously inhibits lipolysis (fat breakdown).

Post-absorptive period (8–12 h postprandial: the so-called fasting phase)

The insulin concentration falls in response to the decline in blood glucose levels, and glucagon becomes the dominant hormone.

Glucagon has two fundamental roles, namely to stimulate the breakdown of glycogen and to assist hepatic gluconeogenesis, i.e. glucose synthesis from non-carbohydrate sources such as amino acids and lactate.

Glycogen is stored with water, so when it is broken down it will also release water, which explains the rapid weight loss observed in early starvation.

Glucagon, in direct opposition to insulin, will also stimulate lipolysis and fat mobilization. It is therefore a catabolic hormone, whilst insulin is a direct antagonist and is anabolic in function. The insulin/glucagon ratio will therefore primarily determine the final metabolic milieu.

Starvation

If starvation extends beyond the normal post-absorptive stage, the glycogen stores in the liver are rapidly depleted within 18 to 24 h to provide glucose for the tissues that require glucose as their mandatory fuel.

Once this supply of glucose has been exhausted, further glucose has to be provided by gluconeogenesis from amino acids in skeletal muscle, glycerol from fat stores and lactate from glucose degradation in red blood cells and the renal medulla. The stimulus for this process is the fall in blood glucose which stimulates the release of glucagon and the reduction in insulin secretion.

As starvation proceeds, skeletal muscle adapts to fat utilization (see Fig. 2.3). In addition to this switch in fuel utilization, the *metabolic rate will fall* (by up to 30 per cent) due to the following:

- a reduction in the mass of metabolically active tissue, i.e. skeletal muscle over a long period of time;
- a reduction in physical activity;
- a decrease in metabolic activity of the remaining body tissue.

All of these processes reduce the rate at which energy stores are utilized, and therefore provide a mechanism by which the body can conserve its stores. In the healthy individual, there are 15 kg of fat reserves. Fat is well placed to fulfil the role of an energy store, as it provides *twice* the energy per gram of protein or carbohydrate. Furthermore, both protein and carbohydrate are stored in association with water, while fat is not. This reduces the energy content of protein and carbohydrate per gram stored in tissue.

It can be calculated from data on hunger strikers that, *in the absence of trauma or complications*, an average 70 kg man will survive for 60–70 days without food.

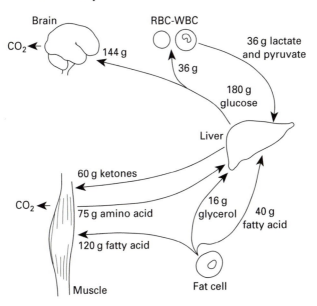

Fig. 2.3 Substrate distribution in fasting humans (adapted from Cahill, G.F. 1970: Starvation in man. *New England Journal of Medicine* **282**, 668–75).

In contrast, in critical illness the hormonal balance is altered by the stress and inflammatory response. The decrease in metabolic rate and protection of skeletal muscle which take place in starvation are not observed and increased proteolysis and lipolysis occur.

Critical illness can also occur in either a previously well-nourished individual or a malnourished individual, and this will affect the overall metabolic response. It is important to note that the effect of critical illness coupled with malnutrition can hasten the catabolic effect.

The metabolic response to injury/trauma

The metabolic response to injury has evolved as a means whereby the body can improve outcome after mild to moderate trauma.

However, even if maintenance or excessive quantities of nutrition are provided, catabolism will only be minimized when the factors responsible for the catabolism are identified and treated. This is because of the influence of hormones and cytokines which are produced in response to the insult.

In the critically ill patient, the distinguishing feature is the hypermetabolic response to the insult. This response can include:

- an alteration in energy needs and production;
- preferential catabolism of body glucose, fat and protein stores;
- limitation of intake by anorexia;
- decreased intestinal absorption if the gut is poorly perfused;
- production of immune cells and acute-phase hepatic proteins;
- fever (if infection is present);
- sodium and fluid retention due to the influence of hormones and oxidative stress.

The degree of hypermetabolism is proportional to the severity of the injury, and is influenced by the type of injury (see Fig. 2.4).

The pattern of clinical response after injury, i.e. the phases of ebb, flow and anabolism, is no longer as simplistic as the model suggested by Cuthbertson in 1932. Neither is the rise in energy expenditure considered to be as excessive as was previously thought. This is partly due to improvements in nursing practice and intensive care support modalities.

A number of responses have been identified in the metabolic response to injury of shock, resuscitation, systemic inflammatory

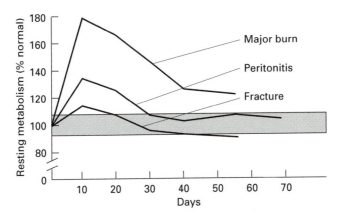

Fig. 2.4 The quantitative metabolic responses with varying types of severity of injury (adapted from Zaloga, G. 1994: *Nutrition in critical care*. St Louis: Mosby.

response (SIRS), organ dysfunction/failure and recovery/death. These phases do not always follow this sequence, and indeed some of these phases *may not occur at all* in the progression of the illness.

Box 2.1 What is SIRS? (systemic inflammatory response syndrome)

Definition: The systemic inflammatory response to a variety of severe clinical insults, i.e. sepsis.
The response is manifested by two or more of the following conditions:

- temperature > 38°C or < 36°C;
- heart rate > 90 beats/min;
- respiratory rate > 20 breaths/min;
- WBC > 12 000 or < 4000 cells/mm^3 or > 10% immature neutrophils;
- PCO_2 < 32 mmHg (< 4.3 kPa) with hyperventilation.

Note: Non-infectious processes, e.g pancreatitis, haemorrhage and tissue injury, can also result in SIRS.

Common initiating events for the hypermetabolic response include:

- septic shock;
- perfusion deficit, e.g. haemorrhage, low cardiac output;
- inflammation, e.g. pancreatitis;
- necrotic tissue, e.g. post trauma, arterial embolus.

Both sepsis and organ hypoperfusion can induce an inflammatory response.

Box 2.2 What is sepsis?

Definition: The systemic response to infection. The term is confined to those conditions in which the cause of SIRS is infection.

Box 2.3 What is infection?

Definition: Microbial phenomenon characterized by an inflammatory response to the presence of micro-organisms or the invasion of normally sterile host tissue by those organisms.

Box 2.4 What is septic shock?

Definition: Sepsis with hypotension, despite adequate fluid resuscitation, together with the presence of perfusion abnormalities that may include, but are not limited to, lactic acidosis, oliguria, or an acute alteration in mental status. Patients who are on vasopressors, e.g. nitroprusside, may not be hypotensive at the time when perfusion abnormalities are measured.

If the patient survives the initial injury, a number of response patterns can emerge:

A stable post-resuscitative hypermetabolic phase – the systemic inflammatory response syndrome (SIRS) – can lead to a progressive multiple organ dysfunction syndrome (MODS) or to a recovery phase. MODS can be fatal.

Box 2.5 What is MODS? (multiple organ dysfunction syndrome)

Definition: The presence of altered organ function in an acutely ill patient such that homeostasis cannot be maintained without intervention. Infection is probably the most common single cause of development of MODS.

The role of hormones and cytokines

The hypermetabolic response is thought to maximize a healing response to injury. Wounds have a high requirement, primarily for oxygen and glucose, due to rapid cell multiplication, and therefore the hormonal response is aimed at producing an adequate supply of both. In order to meet this need, catabolism of stored fuels (fats, proteins and glycogen) occurs.

Unlike the situation in starvation, this catabolism is partly mediated by the counter-regulatory hormones, so called because their effects are opposite to those of insulin (see Fig. 2.5). These include adrenocorticotrophic hormone (ACTH), growth hormone, catecholamines, cortisol and glucagon, and their release is stimulated by the increased activity of the sympathetic nervous system.

These hormones maintain the supply of glucose and result in hyperglycaemia. Their goal is to provide energy and precursors to maintain the metabolic and immunological response. However, unlike starvation, insulin is present in increased quantities but many tissues are resistant to its action, especially skeletal muscle (so-called *insulin resistance*).

In addition to the hormonal response, the invasion of pathogens and the injury itself will activate the immune system to elicit widespread metabolic changes. Immune function is also dependent on glucose and increased liver production of acute-phase proteins as part of the generalized immune response. The acute-phase proteins have been defined as those plasma proteins which increase by 25 per cent or more in the first 7 days following tissue damage. These include C-reactive protein, alpha-acid glycoprotein, caeruloplasmin and alpha-1 antitrypsin. The clinical importance of these proteins has yet to be fully elucidated. However, it is speculated that they are involved in the processes of inflammation and tissue repair.

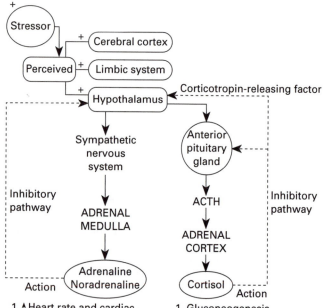

Fig. 2.5 Stress, the hormonal response. (From Adam, S. and Osborne, S., *Nursing Science and Critical Care Practice*, Oxford University Press.)

This altered hepatic protein synthesis in response to injury has been shown to occur at the expense of the other nutritional carrier proteins, namely albumin and transferrin. Therefore, while the concentrations of acute-phase proteins are rising, the plasma concentrations of albumin and transferrin decrease *and are independent of nutritional status.*

NOTE: *Albumin is therefore not a good indicator of nutritional status* (see Chapter 3).

The main aims of the immune response are:

- to disadvantage and destroy invading pathogens;
- to repair damaged tissues;
- to restore tissue function to normal.

This activation leads to the production of the following mediators:

- immunoglobulins;
- complement proteins;
- cytokines.

Immunoglobulins are plasma proteins synthesized by plasma cells and lymphocytes. They are produced in response to a previously known antigen.

Complement proteins are found in serum and serve as antimicrobial factors in host defence.

Cytokines are a large group of proteins and peptides which are involved in signalling between cells of the immune system and include:

- interleukins;
- bradykinin;
- interferons;
- colony-stimulating factors;
- tumour necrosis factor (TNF);
- transforming growth factors.

There are at least three specific cytokines which not only mediate and modulate immune system activity but also cause widespread metabolic changes. These are interleukin 1 (IL-1), interleukin 6 (IL-6) and TNF.

These cytokines belong to a subgroup of cytokines called pro-inflammatory cytokines, which are the key mediators in inflammation. Once produced, IL-1 and TNF can stimulate the production of the other cytokines and also of IL-6, thereby initiating cascades of pro-inflammatory cytokines and other inflammatory mediators.

Oxidants and oxidant-free radical donors, nitric oxide, hydrogen peroxide and superoxide radicals are produced by phagocytes, and also by ischaemia-reperfusion injury, which further enhance cytokine production.

The effects of cytokines and hormones in stress are summarized in Fig. 2.6.

In malnourished patients, who have a reduced ability to produce cytokines, the prognosis is poor because these patients are unable to generate a hostile environment for pathogens.

These widespread metabolic changes:

- facilitate the delivery of nutrients to the immune system;
- assist in the repair of tissues;
- control cytokine production;
- protect healthy tissues from the effects of free radicals and other oxidant molecules;
- remove from the bloodstream nutrients that may assist pathogen multiplication.

The mechanisms underlying these metabolic changes are complex and involve the interaction between cytokines, the hypothalamus and the direct effect of IL-1 and TNF on peripheral tissues.

Increased activity of the sympathetic nervous system promotes increased production of glucocorticoids and catecholamines.

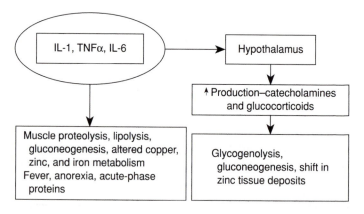

Fig. 2.6 The effects of cytokines and hormones in the stress response.

- *Glucocorticoids* are steroids, e.g. glucagon, which are secreted by the pancreas in response to changes in blood glucose concentrations.
- *Catecholamines*, e.g. adrenaline and noradrenaline, are secreted by the adrenal medulla and sympathetic nervous system in response to stress.

Catecholamines, glucocorticoids and cytokines enhance glycogen breakdown and gluconeogenesis. The cytokines also stimulate production of corticotrophin-releasing factor by their action on the central nervous system. IL-1, TNF and also factors such as hypoxia and sepsis, which induce production of these cytokines, stimulate skeletal muscle catabolism.

However, excessive or inappropriate production of cytokines has been associated with morbidity and mortality in a number of conditions where the immune system has been activated, e.g. sepsis, respiratory distress syndrome, systemic lupus erythematosus and inflammatory bowel disease (Fig. 2.7).

In general, however, many of the responses to stress/trauma are beneficial to the patient. These also include tissue uptake of minerals and trace elements, especially iron, which can slow bacterial growth. Moreover, anorexia and malaise occur to reduce the energy demands of the gut and skeletal muscle so that energy can be directed more appropriately to the immune and repair responses.

The role of nutrition provision in the critically ill

Why feed?

In 1994, Hill reported the measurement of changes in muscle mass in 10 multiple injury patients (mean ISS = 34). He found over a 21-day period an average loss of 17 per cent in total body stores, of which 70 per cent came from skeletal muscle. Potentially this could have the following effects:

Decreased muscle strength: muscle fatigues occurring more readily and muscle relaxation is delayed, with a possible delay in mobilization post-surgery.

Such deterioration in muscle function has been observed after 2 weeks of malnutrition, before any changes in conventional indices of nutritional assessment (Jeejeebhoy, 1988).

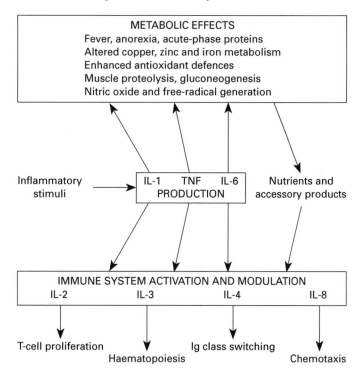

Fig. 2.7 Influence of pro-inflammatory cytokines upon the immune system and metabolism after invasion of the host by pathogens (adapted from Grimble, R.F. 1996: Interaction between nutrients, pro-inflammatory cytokines and inflammation. *Clinical Science* **91**, 122).

Arora and Rochester (1982) have also demonstrated that respiratory muscle strength and maximum voluntary ventilation were significantly reduced in 16 malnourished patients without respiratory disease.

Since the purpose of nutritional support in the critically ill is maintenance rather than repletion, any substrates given in excess of requirements will necessitate more work for the body. This will involve oxidation and storage processes, and measurements of the oxygen consumed and the carbon dioxide produced may be used to estimate the optimal energy intake in the unfed state.

The ratio of carbon dioxide produced to oxygen consumed is defined as the *respiratory quotient* (RQ).

Box 2.6 Respiratory quotients

Fuel	RQ
Carbohydrate	1.00
Fat	0.7
Protein	0.81
Alcohol	0.67

An RQ of 0.85 indicates that equal amounts of protein, fat and carbohydrate (glucose) are being metabolized.

The provision of excess calories as glucose will increase the RQ to > 1.00, which will favour an increase in carbon dioxide production and retention, and hence more difficulty in weaning off the ventilator.

Excess carbohydrate (given as glucose, for example) will cause the following:

- steatosis of the liver.
  Excess glucose (i.e. beyond the body's ability to oxidize for energy) is initially converted to glycogen. However, when stores are replete (about 400 g), the excess is converted to fat, because this entails extra metabolic work with associated carbon dioxide production;
- hyperglycaemia – exacerbated by insulin resistance;
- delayed weaning off the ventilator, since more respiratory work is involved in clearing the carbon dioxide generated by lipogenesis.

Excess fat provided as > 50 per cent of total calories:

- overloads the reticulo-endothelial system (RES). There is an increase in hydrolysis of triglycerides and release of glycerol and free fatty acids which reduces RES clearance rates.
- impairs alveolar gas exchange. Lipids may become deposited in the lungs and impair diffusion of gases.

Excess protein provision *increases the rate of protein synthesis and breakdown* with no improvement in overall balance.

Energy and protein intakes should therefore just meet requirements, or else should be slightly underestimated, to avoid overfeeding.

Nutrient modulation in the critically ill

There is now a wide range of feeds for the critically ill, supplemented with specific nutrients which are marketed as conferring a number of benefits to the patient. These include enhancement of immune function and preservation of skeletal muscle mass, to name just two.

The following discussion will detail the rationale for their inclusion in feeds. For information on the specific feeds and the clinical evidence to support their use see Chapter 5.

Fats

Fats (lipids) are essential constituents of cell membranes. The fluidity of these membranes is influenced by dietary lipids. Any alteration in the fluidity of cell membranes could change the avidity with which cytokines bind to receptors, thereby influencing their activity.

Lipids rich in omega-3 polyunsaturated fatty acids (PUFA) appear to reduce responsiveness to cytokines. These include the long-chain fatty acids, eicosapentaenoic and docosahexaenoic acids, and are found mainly in fish oils.

Other putative advantages of these PUFAs include the following:

- reduced thromboxane production;
- increased prostaglandin synthesis (thromboxane and prostaglandins are inflammatory mediators synthesized from lipids);
- a reduced vasospastic response to catecholamines;
- reduced blood viscosity;
- possible resistance to toxic factors.

It is possible that future lipid profiles in both enteral and parenteral feeds could enhance lung function by improving membrane composition, changing the pattern of prostaglandin synthesis or enhancing surfactant production.

Medium-chain triglycerides (MCTs)

These fats do not require carnitine for their transport into mitochondria. They are also water soluble, and do not require bile salts for dispersal. They travel primarily via the portal circulation to the liver, bypassing the lymphatic system. MCTs are therefore more rapidly hydrolysed than long-chain triglycerides (see Fig. 2.8).

The advantage of this is that these fats can be rapidly cleared from the plasma, thereby reducing hyperlipidaemia and hepatic steatosis. Furthermore, the reticulo-endothelial system shows minimal uptake and therefore the provision of fat as MCTs may lead to less impairment of the RES if supplied intravenously.

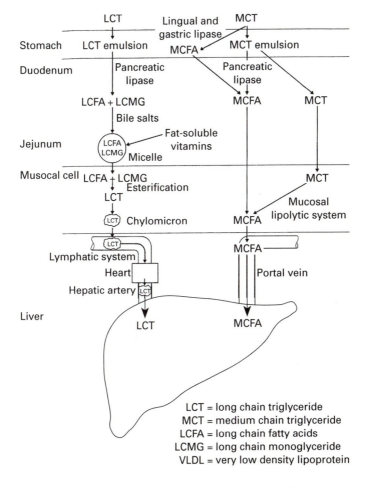

Fig. 2.8 Absorption and metabolism of long-chain and medium-chain tri-glycerides (adapted from Linder, M.C. (ed.) 1991: *Nutritional bichemistry and metabolism with clinical applications*, 2nd edn. Amsterdam: Elsevier).

The principal sources of MCTs are coconut and palm kernel oils.

Short-chain fatty acids (SCFAs) e.g. butyrate, acetate and propionate

SCFAs are primarily the products of fermentation of dietary fibre, which takes place mainly in the colonocytes (cells of the colon), and can supply up to 5 to 10 per cent of daily energy requirements.

SCFAs also benefit the patient by stimulating increased colonic blood flow, promoting salt and water absorption, and stimulating mucosal proliferation.

Amino acids

Glutamine

Glutamine is an amino acid which appears to become conditionally essential after major trauma/stress. It has therefore been suggested that current feeds contain inadequate quantities of glutamine under these conditions.

The properties of glutamine are as follows.

- It is the most abundant free amino acid in the blood and amino acid pool.
- It is the principal fuel for rapidly dividing cells of the small intestine and immune system, e.g. enterocytes, lymphocytes.
- It is a precursor of nucleotides, i.e. DNA and RNA.
- It is a trophic factor for the maintenance of the gut mucosa.

Glutamine is used preferentially as a fuel by the gut in critical illness.

Arginine

Like glutamine, arginine is a conditionally essential amino acid which has an immunomodulating effect.

The properties of arginine are as follows.

- It is a substrate precursor for nitric oxide production (nitric oxide has been implicated in a wide range of immunological and vasoactive functions).

- It is used by all tissues as a substrate for cytoplasmic and nuclear protein synthesis.
- It is essential for ammonia detoxification by urea synthesis.

Nucleotides

The properties of nucleotides are as follows.

- They are precursors of DNA and RNA.
- They increase protein synthesis.
- They are involved in the regulation of several T-cell-mediated immune responses.

Rapidly dividing cells, e.g. T-lymphocytes and intestinal epithelial cells, have a limited ability to synthesize nucleotides during malnutrition and in periods of rapid growth, such as inflammation. This indicates that there may be a need for supplementation in conditions of stress.

Branched-chain amino acids (BCAAs), e.g. valine, leucine and isoleucine

BCAAs compete with aromatic amino acids (phenylalanine, tyrosine and tryptophan) for entry to the brain.

In patients with liver disease, the provision of up to three times the quantity of BCAAs to aromatic amino acids is speculated to reduce the availability of aromatic amino acids which, in excess, can cause impairment of neurotransmitter synthesis that may promote the development of encephalopathy. The results of this type of treatment have been variable, and BCAAs are therefore not used routinely for feeding these types of patients.

The production of cytokines, acute-phase proteins and glutathione (a tripeptide consisting of the three amino acids glycine, glutamic acid and cysteine) is influenced by the adequacy of intake of both protein and the sulphur-containing amino acids methionine and cysteine.

Glutathione protects tissues from free radical injury, and is necessary for lymphocyte proliferation and macrophage function.

It has been estimated that, during major infection, the amount of protein required to produce and maintain an increase in circulating leucocytes and acute-phase proteins is 45 g daily (see Chapter 3 for protein requirements).

Why is nutritional support important in the critically ill?

The sequence of events described above leads to severe wasting and loss of body stores within a very short space of time. When malnutrition is superimposed on trauma, the modulating effects of starvation are lost and the catabolic effects are enhanced.

The primary purpose of providing nutritional support must therefore be *to provide sufficient energy to spare protein*. About 1 g/kg actual body weight will reduce skeletal muscle catabolism, but a significant proportion will be used to support immunological and hepatic synthesis and for healing wounds.

Nutritional support should therefore always commence as early as possible in order to achieve this and avoid further complications.

Table 2.2 A comparison of the responses to starvation and injury in man

Characteristic finding	Starvation	Metabolic response to injury
Energy needs	Decreased	Increased
Primary fuel (RQ)	Fat (0.75)	Mixed (0.85)
Insulin	Decreased	Increased (resistance)
Ketones	Present	Absent
Counter-regulatory hormones	Basal	Increased
Cytokines	Basal	Increased
Total body water	Decreased	Increased
Proteolysis	Decreased	Accelerated
Glycogenolysis	Increased	Accelerated
Body Stores		
Skeletal muscle	Reduced	Reduced
Fat	Reduced	Reduced
Visceral protein	Preserved	Increased (liver immune)
Weight loss	Gradual	Accelerated

(adapted from Daley, B.J. and Bistrain, B.R. 1994: *Nutritional assessment*. In: Zaloga, G.P. (ed.), *Nutrition in critical care*. 1994: Mosby, St Louis, MO: 13.

Case study

Mrs Douglas is a slightly overweight 35-year-old who presented to A&E complaining of a one-week history of general malaise, pyrexia and a chest infection. She was prescribed antibiotics by her GP, but her condition deteriorated, and she became increasingly breathless.

On admission, she had a reduced arterial O_2 saturation, and her increasing distress necessitated endotracheal intubation and ventilation.

Diagnosis: community-acquired pneumonia.

The patient was nil by mouth for 7 days on 2.5 L of dextrose saline (400 kcal/day) due to suspected ileus and the ICU team's belief that she was responding well to treatment.

She was extubated on day 8 and her recovery was uneventful except for the fact that she sustained a large weight loss of 5.6 kg (~11 lb) after 10 days on the ICU.

Her oral intake after extubation was ~500 kcal daily, an intake with which she was pleased as she wants to lose weight.

On discharge from hospital she continues on a low-calorie diet, but to her dismay gains weight at a rate of 0.2 kg per day (~0.5 lb). *Why has she gained weight?*

Mrs Douglas received an inadequate supply of essential glucose for her mandatory glucose-requiring tissues, specifically the brain.

She therefore had to use alternative energy stores to supply the glucose, which would have been glycogen in the first instance, and then protein. The weight loss she experienced on ICU was due to loss of a combination of fat and intracellular water, as glycogen and protein are stored with water.

On resumption of her normal level of activity, on a low-energy diet, fat would be oxidized preferentially.

Carbohydrate and protein reserves are replaced last in the recovery phase, and therefore there will be a gain in intracellular water, which will be represented by a weight gain.

References

Arora, N.S. and Rochester, D.F. 1982: Respiratory muscle strength in maximal voluntary ventilation in undernourished patients. *American Review of Respiratory Diseases* **126**, 1265–8.

Cahill, G.F. Jr 1970: Starvation in man. *New England Journal of Medicine* **282**, 668–75.

Cuthbertson, D.P. 1932: Observation on the disturbance of metabolism produced by injury to the limbs. *Quarterly Journal of Medicine* **25**, 233–46.

Hill, G.L. 1994: Impact of nutritional support on the clinical outcome of the surgical patient. *Clinical Nutrition* **13**, 331–40.

Jeejeebhoy, K.N. 1988: Bulk or bounce – the object of nutritional support. *Journal of Parenteral and Enteral Nutrition* **12**, 539–45.

Weissman, C. Kemper, M. and Damask, M.C. 1984: Effect of routine intensive care interaction on metabolic rate. *Chest* **86**, 815–18.

Further reading

American College of Chest Physicians/Society of Critical Care Medicine Consensus Conference Committee, 1992: Definitions for sepsis and organ failure and guidelines for the use of innovative therapies in sepsis. *Critical Care Medicine* **20**, 864–74.

Brittenden, J., Heys, S.D., Ross, J., Park, K.G.M. and Eremin, O. 1994: Nutritional pharmacology: effects of L-arginine on host defences, response to trauma and tumour growth. *Clinical Science* **86**, 123–32.

Chandra, R.J. 1993: Nutrition and the immune system. *Proceedings of the Nutrition Society* **52**, 77–84.

Elia, M. 1995: Changing concepts of nutrient requirements in disease: implications for artificial nutrition support. *Lancet* **345**, 1279–84.

Grimble Robert, F. 1996: Interaction between nutrients, proinflammatory cytokines and inflammation. *Clinical Science* **91**, 121–30.

Kinsella, J.E. 1990: Dietary polyunsaturated fatty acids and eicosanoids. Potential effects on the modulation of inflammatory mediators and immune cells. an overview. *Nutrition* **6**, 24–44.

O'Leary, M.J. and Coakley, J.H. 1996: Nutrition and immunonutrition. *British Journal of Anaesthesia* **77**, 118–27.

Souba, W.W. 1990: Glutamine nutrition: theoretical considerations and therapeutic impact. *Journal of Parenteral and Enteral Nutrition* **14**, 237s–243s.

3

Nutritional assessment of requirements

The aims of this chapter are:

- to define malnutrition and its incidence in patients in UK hospitals;
- to describe the objectives of nutritional assessment;
- to define macronutrient requirements and assessment methods;
- to describe the body compartment model and methods of assessment;
- to describe nutritional parameters commonly used in practice and prediction formulae;
- to define micronutrient requirements and assessment methods.

Malnutrition

Clinically relevant malnutrition has been defined as the state of altered nutritional status that is associated with an increased risk of adverse clinical events, such as complications or death.

The most common form of malnutrition that occurs in the clinical setting is protein energy malnutrition (PEM), which is a reflection of an inadequate protein and energy intake.

The incidence of malnutrition is reported to be as high as 40 per cent in medical and surgical wards in the UK (McWhirter and Pennington, 1994). These figures obviously have a bearing on the nutritional status of those patients who are transferred from such wards to the ICU.

In 1996 Giner *et al.* identified 43 per cent of 129 patients admitted to an ICU as malnourished. Furthermore, the incidence of complications was higher in the malnourished group, and the impact of malnutrition was also greater in the patients who were less ill.

Assessment of the patient on admission to the ICU is therefore crucial for the following reasons:

- to determine the nutritional status of the patient;
- to identify the type and extent of any pre-existing malnutrition;
- to determine the optimal route for artificial nutrition;
- to record a baseline from which changes in the nutritional status of the patient and the efficacy of nutritional support can be evaluated.

Nutrition assessment methods

There is a number of assessment methods developed for research purposes, which are impractical and of little use in the clinical setting. For the purpose of this text they will be excluded. Instead, emphasis will be placed on those practical methods that are used routinely. However, it cannot be over-emphasized that there is **no one** foolproof method of nutrition assessment.

Objective nutritional parameters based on quantitative criteria continue to be used and abused, and there is no consensus on the best nutritional markers. There is no substitute for an experienced common-sense team approach which also takes into consideration the other non-nutritional factors which affect patient outcome, e.g. organ dysfunction and sepsis.

The ability to recover from illness/trauma is only partly dependent on nutritional status, and nutritional support is only one factor affecting outcome. It is also of varying importance in different patients.

Factors affecting nutritional intake

Assessment of requirements will initially involve a physical examination of the patient, accompanied by a review of the patient's history.

The following factors need to be considered:

Previous nutrient intake

- actual intake;
- anorexia;
- excess alcohol intake;

- gastrointestinal tract malfunction affecting intake, digestion or absorption.

Underlying pathology with nutritional effects

- chronic infections or inflammatory states;
- neoplasia;
- endocrine disorders;
- chronic illnesses – pulmonary disease, cirrhosis, or renal failure.

End-organ effects

- oedema/ascites;
- weight changes;
- obesity;
- muscle mass relative to exercise status.

Miscellaneous

- catabolic medications or therapies: steroids, immunosuppressive agents, radiation or chemotherapy;
- pain;
- genetic background;
- other medications – diuretics, laxatives, vitamin and mineral supplements;
- food allergies – food intolerances.

Macronutrient requirements

The macronutrients are carbohydrates and fats (the energy providers) and proteins are the anabolic substrates. Their physiological effect depends on the absolute and relative amounts given and the subject to whom they are administered.

Energy requirements

Energy intake can be determined by measuring the energy produced from the oxidation of carbohydrate, fat and protein (see Table 3.1) and the efficiency of digestion and absorption. If the individual is in energy balance, then intake should be equal to expenditure.

Table 3.1 Energy values for the oxidation of macronutrients

Macronutrient	Energy value (kcal/g)
Carbohydrate	3.75
Protein	4.0
Fat	9.0
Medium-chain triglycerides	8.4
Alcohol	7.0

Total energy expenditure (TEE) consists of three variables (see Chapter 2):

- basal metabolic rate;
- metabolic requirements of activity;
- thermic effects of food or postprandial thermogenesis.

The actual value of postprandial thermogenesis depends on the substrate, i.e. whether it is fat, carbohydrate or protein.

For a mixed diet, a value of 10 per cent is generally assumed. However, if the intake is modest, or if the patient is very malnourished, the contribution to TEE is negligible. Moreover, this value may be significantly less in the critically ill patient receiving long-term parenteral nutrition (Forsberg *et al.*, 1993).

The only other factor left to consider is the effect of activity. This is of minimal significance in the critically ill except when the patient is self-ventilating and tachypnoeic or severely agitated.

In practice, as already mentioned, the RMR can be measured directly as an estimate of total energy requirements. The most accurate practical method is that of indirect calorimetry, which measures the gas exchange, i.e. oxygen uptake and (VO_2) and carbon dioxide release (VCO_2).

Respiratory quotient (RQ) = ratio of O_2 consumed/CO_2 released.

Since the amount of CO_2 released from the combustion of carbohydrate, fat and protein will be different, a precise value for energy expenditure can be obtained by including urinary nitrogen excretion (which reflects protein oxidation). However, in practice this is unnecessary, as the assumption that RQ represents non-protein metabolism creates only a 2 per cent error (Bursztein *et al.*, 1989).

Energy expenditure (EE) can therefore be calculated from the following equation:

$$EE = 3.91 \ VO_2 + 1.10 \ VCO_2 - 1.93 \ N_2$$

(where VO_2 and VCO_2 are expressed in L/min and N_2 is expressed in g/min).

Measurement of VO_2 and VCO_2 is commonly achieved on the ICU using a metabolic cart which will sample all the expiratory gases of the patient and, from VO_2 and VCO_2 will estimate the RQ and energy expenditure and consumption. However, even this method requires a skilled operator, and has limitations in that for a fractionated inspired oxygen concentration (FiO_2) of >60 per cent, it becomes inaccurate.

Energy requirements in such situations need to be calculated using formulae, which also have their drawbacks in that the basal metabolic rate is calculated and add-on factors are used at the discretion of the dietitian.

Previously, the Harris Benedict formula was used extensively, but this formula has a number of disadvantages.

- It was derived from TEE measured in *healthy* individuals, rather than BMR.
- The age range used was narrow, with very few subjects over 55 years of age.
- Few of the subjects were outside the normal range of weight for height.

The most commonly used prediction formula is that of Schofield (1985) (see Appendix 3.1). Alternatively, the Elia nomogram (1990) (see Appendix 3.2) can be used to incorporate changes in metabolic rate depending on the clinical condition.

In critically ill patients, additional factors for weight increase and activity should *NOT* be included until convalescence on a general ward, as these patients cannot use excess energy for weight gain. Inactive patients will use excess energy for fat deposition (see Chapter 2).

Factors to consider when calculating energy expenditure include:

- the patient's age and sex;
- diagnosis and severity of illness;
- conscious level, e.g. Glasgow coma score;
- nutritional intake, e.g. patient fasted/fed/hyperalimentation;
- drugs, e.g. muscle relaxants and sedatives can decrease TEE, and catecholamines can increase TEE. Propofol, a muscle relaxant, provides 1 kcal/mL and needs to be taken into account when calculating energy requirements.

Protein requirements

The data on protein requirements in humans focuses on the minimal amounts required to achieve balance.

Protein requirements can be expressed as grams of nitrogen or protein. The conversion factor is as follows:

1 g of nitrogen = 6.25 g of protein

In the critically ill, the emphasis should be on provision of the optimal amount.

Elwyn (1993) estimated that 14 g of nitrogen daily was sufficient to meet the needs of the moderately stressed patient, and concluded that there was little benefit in providing any nitrogen in excess of this amount.

It should be noted that the goal in these patients is to decrease net protein breakdown, rather than to try to achieve synthesis.

In practice, a quick estimate of requirements for both parenteral and enteral nutrition can be made using the guidelines shown in Boxes 3.1 and 3.2.

Box 3.1 Estimation of energy requirements per kg actual body weight/day

Septic and SIRS	30–35 kcal
Non-septic and SIRS	25–30 kcal

Box 3.2 Estimation of nitrogen requirements per kg actual body weight/day (Elia, 1990)

Normal	–	0.17 g
Hypermetabolic	5–25%	0.20 g
	25–50%	0.25 g
	> 50%	0.30 g

Note: *The maximum amount of nitrogen that can be metabolized by any individual is 18 g per day.*

It should also be noted that parenteral nutrition *should ideally never be administered for less than 7 days' duration*, as there is evidence that there is little benefit to the patient (Campos and Meguid, 1992).

Requirements in specific disease states

Energy and protein requirements in liver disease

Protein energy malnutrition is common in patients with chronic liver disease, but not in patients with acute disease.

Protein restriction is not necessary in the majority of patients with liver disease and in fact could be more harmful and lead to protein energy malnutrition.

Oesophageal varices are not necessarily a contraindication to tube feeding.

Table 3.2 XVIII ESPEN Consensus Conference on Nutrition and Liver Disease, September 1996. Recommendation of consensus group: summary of nutritional requirements (adapted from Plauth *et al.*, 1997)

Clinical condition	*Energy (kcal/kg/day)*	*Protein (g/kg/day)*
Compensated cirrhosis	30–40	1–1.2
Complications, inadequate intake, malnutrition	40–45	1.5
Encephalopathy grade I–II	30–40	Transiently 0.5, then 1–1.5
Encephalopathy grade III–IV	30–40	0.5–1.2

The enteral route is preferred, but if this is impossible, it is recommended that energy should be provided by glucose and fat, with fat providing 35–50 per cent of non-protein calories (see Chapter 6). Nitrogen should be provided using conventional amino-acid solutions (see note below) unless otherwise indicated (see Table 3.2).

NOTE: Branched-chain amino acids (BCAAs) may be useful. This is because in chronic liver disease, changes in plasma levels of amino acids are observed, due to abnormalities in lipid and carbohy-drate metabolism.

Elevation of plasma aromatic amino acids (AAAs), i.e. phenyl-alanine, tyrosine and tryptophan, occurs in tandem with a fall in BCAAs, i.e. valine, leucine and isoleucine. Plasma and brain accu-mulation of AAAs may cause severe impairment of brain neuro-transmitter synthesis, which in turn causes hepatic encephalopathy. This decrease in BCAAs, which compete with AAAs for blood–brain transport, contributes greatly to the accumulation of AAAs in the brain.

BCAAs appear to reverse the coma by competing with AAAs for brain entry, or by decreasing the free levels of tyrosine and ammonia. However, long-term use of these BCAA solutions can cause other plasma amino-acid abnormalities, such as a reduction in tyrosine and cysteine levels, and reductions in nitrogen balance have been observed.

Energy and protein requirements in renal failure

Acute renal failure (ARF) occurs in 25 per cent of all patients admitted to the ICU, but only 10 per cent of these cases will require renal replacement therapy.

ARF can be defined as an acute and marked reduction in glomerular filtration rate. Metabolic waste products accumulate, accompanied by an inability to regulate water and mineral balance.

Energy requirements in renal failure are similar to those of other critically ill patients, i.e. 20 per cent above resting energy expenditure, and they can be calculated from formulae or by indirect calorimetry as described previously.

Protein intake in patients with renal failure depends on the rise in plasma urea, the patient's weight, his or her medical condition and the type of renal replacement therapy, if any.

These patients are typically in negative nitrogen balance and display an increased protein turnover, so protein intake should not be restricted. Attempts should be made to match the degree of catabolism with adequate amounts of protein and energy to minimize losses (Table 3.3).

Table 3.3 Energy and protein requirements/kg actual body weight/day

Therapy	*Nutrients*	
	Protein(g)	*Energy (kcal)*
Continuous haemofiltration/ diafiltration dialysis	1.0–1.2	30–35
Intermittent haemodialysis/ haemofiltration/diafiltration	1.0–1.2	30–35
Non-dialysed/filtered (residual renal function, minimal catabolism)	0.55–0.60	30–35

(Adapted from Daugirdas, J.T. and Todal, S.I. 1994: Nutrition. In *Handbook of dialysis*, 2nd edn. Boston: Little Brown.)

Energy and protein requirements in head injury

The elevation of BMR in the acute head-injured patient can be as high as 40 per cent (Ott *et al.*, 1990), and can last up to 2 weeks post-injury, depending on the type of head injury, e.g. intracranial, extracranial or diffuse. Therefore the consensus is to attempt to feed as early as possible. In practice, a combination of pro-kinetic agents, e.g. metoclopramide and cisapride, is used to offset the delayed gastric emptying which is a consequence of the altered neurological state.

Nutritional requirements per kg actual body weight per day are 1.5–2.5 g of nitrogen and a 20–30 per cent increase in energy (kcal) above BMR using formulae (see Appendices 3.1 and 3.2).

Assessment of body composition

For nutritional purposes, body composition analysis is based on the four-compartment model, i.e. protein, water, minerals (the so-called fat-free mass) and body fat (see Fig. 3.1 for body composition). This model necessitates independent analysis of at least three of the compartments, namely protein, water and fat, as they are all affected by nutritional intake.

Assessment of protein status

The body of an average adult human weighing 70 kg contains about 10 to 13 kg of protein, which is widely distributed in different body tissues (see Table 3.4).

Proteins have important structural functions, e.g. collagen in connective tissue, elastin in skin. They also have a regulatory function, e.g. hormones such as insulin, and enzymes such as lipase. In addition, proteins function as specific protein carriers and mediators of the immune response.

The body is unable to store protein, and therefore any protein loss leads to a loss in structural and regulatory function.

The majority of the body protein is found in skeletal muscle (the so-called *somatic protein*), and contributes 30–50 per cent of the total body protein. Skeletal muscle is of particular significance in the critically ill, as it wastes rapidly in disease and malnutrition. For patients who are ventilator dependent, for example, respiratory muscle strength is a major determinant of weaning ability.

Body composition

Lean body mass: that part of the body totally devoid of fat except for essential lipid (about 2%), i.e. body weight minus the weight of adipose tissue

Fat-free mass: (the mass of the body minus all body fat)

Body cell mass: the total mass of cells in the body where oxygen is consumed and carbon dioxide is produced

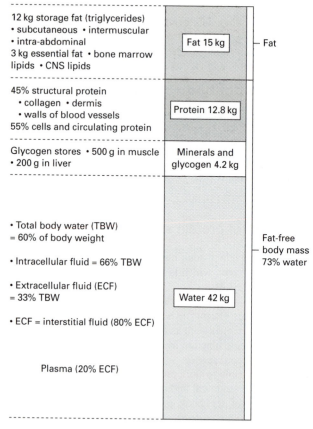

12 kg storage fat (triglycerides)
• subcutaneous • intermuscular
• intra-abdominal
3 kg essential fat • bone marrow
lipids • CNS lipids

Fat 15 kg — Fat

45% structural protein
• collagen • dermis
• walls of blood vessels
55% cells and circulating protein

Protein 12.8 kg

Glycogen stores • 500 g in muscle
• 200 g in liver

Minerals and glycogen 4.2 kg

• Total body water (TBW)
= 60% of body weight

• Intracellular fluid = 66% TBW

• Extracellular fluid (ECF)
= 33% TBW

• ECF = interstitial fluid (80% ECF)

Plasma (20% ECF)

Water 42 kg

Fat-free body mass 73% water

Fig. 3.1 Approximate body compartments of a 74 kg man. (Parenteral and Enteral Group of the British Dietetic Association. 1997: Assessment. In *Pocket guide to clinical nutrition*. Birmingham: British Dietetic Association.)

Table 3.4 The protein content of body tissues

Body tissue	Protein content (g/kg)
Muscle	22
Skeleton	20
Viscera and skin	18
Extracellular	17
Fat	6

The remaining or *visceral protein* consists of serum proteins, erythrocytes, granulocytes and lymphocytes, and is also found in the viscera or organs such as the liver, kidneys, pancreas and heart.

The somatic and visceral protein together comprise the body cell mass, i.e. the metabolically available protein.

The other major protein constituents of the body are found in the non-cellular structural proteins of the cartilage, fibrous and skeletal tissues. To all intents and purposes these can be regarded as fixed in that they are not readily exchangeable with other body pools of protein, and they cannot be mobilized during trauma or stress to counteract any changes in body cell mass that may occur.

Assessment of visceral protein status

Visceral protein status is assessed by the measurement of one or more of the serum proteins listed in Table 3.5.

The visceral protein is the most important compartment in terms of clinical outcome, since the main site for the synthesis of these proteins is the liver, one of the first organs to be affected by protein malnutrition. This is due to the fact that lack of protein substrate will impair the synthesis of serum proteins, resulting in a fall in serum protein concentrations in plasma.

Table 3.5 Serum proteins of hepatic origin

Protein	Half-life	Body pool size (g/kg body weight)
Serum albumin	14–20 days	3–5
Serum transferrin	8–10 days	< 0.1
Serum thyroxine-binding pre-albumin	2–3 days	0.01
Serum retinol-binding protein	12 h	0.002

Table 3.6 Factors affecting serum protein concentrations (adapted from Jeejeebhoy, 1991)

- Inadequate protein intake resulting from: low dietary intakes, anorexia or hypocaloric intravenous infusions
- Altered metabolism generated by: trauma, stress, sepsis and hypoxia
- A specific deficiency of plasma proteins caused by protein-losing enteropathies or liver disease
- Reduced protein synthesis resulting from inadequate energy intake, electrolyte deficiency, trace element deficiencies (e.g. iron and zinc) or vitamin deficiency (e.g. Vitamin A)
- Pregnancy which induces changes in the amount and distribution of body fluids
- Capillary permeability changes
- Use of artificial colloids, causing dilutional decreases in albumin levels
- Altered fluid states

However, on a cautionary note, many non-nutritional factors affect the concentration of serum proteins (Table 3.6). In the critically ill patient, reductions in the levels of many serum proteins occur so frequently as a result of the stress response, that some workers have advocated their use only during convalescence (Carpentier *et al.*, 1982).

Albumin is a classic example of this phenomenon, in that there is a shift of albumin from the intravascular to the extravascular space in the presence of traumatic injury or ongoing stress, resulting in a transient fall in serum albumin levels. This shift could be as much as threefold in patients with septic shock.

Serum proteins that are useful for measuring short-term changes in protein status must have a short-half life (the biological half-life of a protein is the time taken for protein turnover to take place).

The protein must also have a small body pool, a rapid rate of synthesis, and a fairly constant catabolic rate that responds specifically to protein energy deprivation, but is not affected by external factors.

From the following discussion it will become apparent that none of these visceral proteins fulfil all of these criteria.

Serum albumin

Serum albumin concentrations are affected by a number of variables, some of which are listed in Table 3.6. These include age, infection, zinc depletion (causing a decrease) and dehydration (causing an increase due to a reduced plasma volume).

Furthermore, due to its long half-life, it is not very sensitive to any short-term changes in protein status. As more than 50 per cent is present outside the vascular space, serum albumin will reflect changes within the intravascular space, not the total visceral pool.

In addition, any reduction in albumin synthesis in the liver will be compensated for by reduced breakdown. Redistribution of albumin from the extravascular to the intravascular space occurs, and hence the net change in serum albumin levels may be very small.

For instance, Keys *et al.* (1950), in the classical Minnesota experiment, demonstrated that total circulating albumin was reduced by only 2 per cent after 24 weeks of reduced energy and protein intake. There was an associated fall in serum albumin levels of 10 per cent which Keys attributed to other causes. In contrast, in short-term starvation and even in patients with anorexia nervosa, serum albumin levels are usually normal (Broom *et al.*, 1986). Furthermore, Anderson and Wochers (1982) have found that hypoalbuminaemia correlates poorly with nutritional status.

For the above reasons, albumin is therefore not a good indicator of nutritional status. However, it has been shown to be an accurate prognostic indicator of complications and death. A serum albumin concentration *below 35 g/L* reflects a non-specific impairment of the body's ability to cope with major illness, surgical intervention or sepsis. It is for these reasons alone that albumin should be included as a biochemical marker in nutritional assessment.

Hypoalbuminaemia is also closely associated with extracellular fluid expansion, a condition which in itself may have a damaging effect on wound healing, gas transport, and the function of different organs. However, in the vast majority of ICU patients in whom artificial colloids are used, this fluid expansion is not observed.

Other indices of visceral protein status

Serum transferrin has a shorter half-life than albumin, and therefore responds more rapidly to changes in protein status. However, because it is an iron-transport protein, it is markedly affected by changes in iron status, e.g. anaemia, chronic infection, blood transfusions. In addition, a wide range of concentrations has been observed among malnourished subjects, both before and during refeeding (Ingenbleek *et al.*, 1975).

Unfortunately it is also affected by a number of other factors, such as disease state, and is therefore not sensitive enough to be used as a nutritional marker, and in any event it is not routinely measured in the acute setting, as the assay method is time-consuming and expensive.

Serum retinol binding protein and *serum thyroxine binding pre-albumin* have shorter half-lives than serum transferrin, but are of little use in the critically ill, as they are both extremely sensitive to minor changes in inflammation or stress.

Nitrogen balance

This is a measure of net changes in total body protein mass. In total, 90–95 per cent of nitrogen is excreted in the urine, the remainder being lost in stools, skin, hair and nails. Consequently, measurements of urinary nitrogen excretion over a given time period will reflect the state of nitrogen balance.

In practice, urinary urea nitrogen is measured, as urinary nitrogen measurements are time-consuming.

The nitrogen balance is then calculated in the following way. A 24-h urine collection for urea is analysed.

Nitrogen output = urinary urea/mmol/24 h $\times$ 0.033 + obligatory losses + any extra renal losses.

Obligatory losses come from hair, faeces and skin (~ 2–4 g nitrogen/day).

Extra renal losses may include nitrogen losses from sweat, burns exudate, bed sores and fistulae.

Nitrogen balance (g/day) = nitrogen intake − nitrogen output

The drawbacks of this assessment method are that it can be affected by:

- inaccurate 24-h urine collections;
- unaccounted large extra-renal losses;
- fluctuating plasma urea levels;
- resolving haematoma with associated urea production.

Therefore, in practice, changes in total body protein can be monitored indirectly using anthropometric indices, e.g. weight, skin-fold thicknesses and biochemical measurements.

Assessment of fat status

Unfortunately, there is no definitive method for assessment of fat status in the critically ill, and direct measurement of total body fat is still not possible.

However, it is estimated that in order to prevent essential fatty acid deficiency, approximately 3–4.5 per cent of total energy should be provided as fat.

For critically ill patients, requirements are 0.8–1.0 g/kg body weight/day.

Assessment of fluid status

Starvation, stress and refeeding induce profound changes in the patient's fluid status. In the acutely ill patient there is an absolute increase in extracellular fluid.

Recently, however, Finn *et al.* (1996) have demonstrated that the profound loss of body protein which occurs in the critically ill is triggered and maintained by cell shrinkage secondary to cellular dehydration. The proteolysis associated with this phenomenon can be associated with poor wound healing, immune dysfunction and impaired organ function.

Currently, assessment of fluid status can be determined from a combination of clinical examination, central venous pressure (CVP), Doppler ultrasound, plasma and urinary electrolytes, and fluid balance measurements.

Conversely, fluid overload can have a number of serious sequelae and therefore needs to be assessed carefully before determining the given volume of any artificial nutrition.

In addition, it is important to consider not only the volume but also the electrolyte content of any fluid losses (an example is given in Appendix 3.3).

It should also be noted that artificial nutrition in itself can induce changes in body water distribution.

Electrolyte requirements

Oral and intravenous electrolyte requirements are summarized in Table 3.7.

Table 3.7 Electrolyte requirements

Electrolyte	Oral	Intravenous
Sodium	60–100 mmol/day, 1 mmol/kg	1–1.5 mmol/kg/24 h
Potassium	50–100 mmol/day, 1 mmol/kg	1 mmol/kg/24 h or 5 mmol/g N_2 if serum K is < 3.5 mmol/L
Chloride	60–100 mmol/24 h	1–1.5 mmol/kg

(Parenteral and Enteral Group of the British Dietetic Association. 1997: Requirements. In *Pocket guide to clinical nutrition*. Birmingham: British Dietetic Association.)

Box 3.3 Tests used most frequently as functional indices of nutritional status

Anthropometric measurements
  Weight (kg)
  Usual weight (kg)
  Ideal body weight (kg)
  Height (m)
  Percentage weight loss, if applicable (%)

Arm circumference (cm)

Biochemical indices

Plasma electrolytes, e.g. sodium, potassium
  Magnesium
  Calcium
  Phosphorus
  Urea
  Creatinine
  24-h urinary urea

Previous diet and nutrition status (if available)

Protein intake
  Energy intake
  Current resting energy expenditure (measured or calculated from formulae) (see Appendices 3.1 and 3.2)

Micronutrient requirements

For the purposes of this discussion, micronutrients refers to vitamins, minerals and trace elements.

Micronutrients perform two distinct functions. They act as cofactors or coenzymes in a variety of enzyme-catalysed reactions, and they participate in free-radical-scavenging mechanisms.

Free radicals are substances (e.g. superoxide, hydroxyl, hydroperoxy) which contain unpaired electrons and have the potential to cause serious chemical damage due to their high chemical reactivity. This process is called oxidative metabolism, and the micronutrients therefore function as antioxidants.

The main oxidative damage is to the polyunsaturated fatty acid components of membrane structures.

In the catabolic state, oxidative metabolism increases, and the free-radical scavengers can protect tissues against this damage. For example, vitamins C and E and beta-carotene are important antioxidants.

The effects of critical illness on micronutrient requirements are as follows:

- an increase in the requirement for micronutrients, associated with the increase in metabolic rate;
- reduced absorption of micronutrients due, for example, to short gut, loss of integrity of intestinal mucosa, delayed gastric emptying;
- increased losses of micronutrients due to diarrhoea, fistulae losses, dialysis, nasogastric aspirates.

Most enteral and parenteral formulae allow for these increases by providing micronutrients in excess of requirements. However, there will be certain conditions in which patients may still require additional amounts, e.g. severe burns, where additional micronutrients may be required.

The particular requirements in these specific disease states will therefore now be considered.

Severe burns, i.e. > 30 per cent of total body surface area

- Consider vitamin C, trace elements, and iron. In practice, usual doses of vitamin C should not exceed 1 g/day. Zinc should not be supplemented routinely as there are losses of all trace elements in burn exudate. Intravenous trace element supplementation may be of benefit in improving immune responses after burn injury. If there are large blood losses, patients tend to be transfused and therefore iron supplementation is unecessary.

Patients undergoing intermittent or continuous dialysis or haemofiltration

- Consider water-soluble vitamins, e.g. thiamine, pyridoxine, folic acid.
- Consider vitamin C and zinc.
- Consider calcium and phosphorus.
- All dialysis patients should receive daily supplementary folic acid and B vitamins.

Table 3.8 Daily vitamin/mineral requirements in renal failure

Vitamin/mineral	Daily requirement
Folic acid	1 mg
Thiamine (vitamin B_1)	30 mg
Pyridoxine	20 mg
Other B vitamins	Usual DRV
Zinc	20 mg
Avoid vitamin A	

(Adapted from Daugirdas, J.T. and Todal, S.I. 1994: Nutrition. In *Handbook of dialysis*, 2nd edn. Boston: Little Brown.)

Table 3.9 Daily vitamin requirements in enteral and parenteral nutrition

Vitamin	Enteral nutrition	Parenteral nutrition
Thiamine (mg)	0.8–1.1	3–20
Riboflavin (mg)	1.1–1.3	3–8
Niacin (mg)	2–18	40
Pyridoxine (mg)	1.2–2.0	4.0–6.0
Folate (μg)	200–400	200–400
Vitamin B_{12} (μg)	1.5–3.0	5–15
Pantothenic acid (mg)	3–7	10–20
Biotin (μg)	10–200	60
Vitamin A (μg)	600–1200	800–2500
Vitamin C (mg)	40–60	100
Vitamin D (μg)	5	5
Vitamin K (μg/kg)	1	0.03–1.5
Vitamin E (mg)	10	10

(Parenteral and Enteral Group of the British Dietetic Association. 1997: Requirements. In *Pocket guide to clinical nutrition*. Birmingham: British Dietetic Association.)

Table 3.10 Daily trace element requirements in enteral and parenteral nutrition

Element	Enteral nutrition (μmol)	Parenteral nutrition (μmol)
Zinc	110–145	145
Copper	16–20	20
Iodine	1–1.2	1.0
Manganese	30–60	5–10
Fluoride	95–150	50
Chromium	0.5–1.0	0.2–0.4
Selenium	0.8–0.9	0.25–0.5
Molybdenum	0.5–4.0	0.2–1.2

(Parenteral and Enteral Group of the British Dietetic Association. 1997: Requirements. In *Pocket guide to clinical nutrition*. Birmingham: British Dietetic Association.)

Table 3.11 Daily mineral requirements in enteral and parenteral nutrition

Mineral	Enteral nutrition	Parenteral nutrition
Calcium	20 mmol/24 h, 0.2 mmol/kg	0.1–0.15 mmol/kg/24h
Magnesium	12–14 mmol/24h, 0.2 mmol/kg	0.1–0.2 mmol/kg/24h
Phosphate*	25 mmol/24h, 0.3 mmol/kg	0.5–0.7 mmol/kg/24h

*Do not exceed 50 mmol phosphate/day in enteral or parenteral feeds.
(Parenteral and Enteral Group of the British Dietetic Association. 1997: Requirements. In *Pocket guide to clinical nutrition*. Birmingham: British Dietetic Association.)

References

Anderson, C.F. and Wochers, D.N. 1982: The utility of serum albumin values in the nutritional assessment of hospitalised patients. *Mayo Clinic Proceedings* **57**, 181.

Broom, J., Fraser, M.H., McKensie, K., Miller, J.D.B. and Fleck, A. 1986: The protein metabolic response to short-term starvation in man. *Clinical Nutrition* **5**, 63–5.

Bursztein, S., Saphar, P., Singer, P. and Elwyn, D. 1989: A mathematical analysis of indirect calorimetry measurements in acutely ill patients. *American Journal of Clinical Nutrition* **50**, 227–30.

Campos, A.C.L. and Meguid, M.M. 1992: A critical appraisal of the usefulness of perioperative nutritional support. *American Journal of Clinical Nutrition* **55**, 117–30.

Carpentier, Y.A., Barthel, J. and Bruyns, J. 1982: Plasma protein concentrations in nutritional assessment. *Proceedings of the Nutrition Society* **41**, 405–17.

Elia, M. 1990: Artificial nutrition support. *Medicine International* **82**, 3392–6.

Elywn, D.H. 1993: Protein and energy requirement: effect of clinical state. *Clinical Nutrition* **12** (Suppl. 1), 44–52.

Finn, P.J., Plank, L.D., Clark, M.A., Connolly, A.B. and Hill, G.H. 1996: Progressive cellular dehydration and proteolysis in critically ill patients. *Lancet* **347**, 654–6.

Forsberg, E., Soop, M. and Thorne, A. 1993: Thermogenic response to total parenteral nutrition in depleted patients with multiple organ failure. *Clinical Nutrition* **12**, 253–61.

Giner, M., Laviano, A., Meguid, M.M. and Gleason, J.R. 1996: In 1995 a correlation between malnutrition and poor outcome in critically ill patients still exists. *Nutrition* **12**, 23–9.

Ingenbleek, Y., van den Schrieck, H.G., de Nayer, P.L and De Visscher, M. 1975: Albumin, transferrin and the thyroxine-binding pre-albumin/retinol binding protein (TBPA-RBP) complex in assessment of malnutrition. *Clinica Chimica Acta* **63**, 61–7.

Jeejeebhoy, K.N. 1981: Protein nutrition in clinical practice. *British Medical Bulletin* **37**, 11–17.

Keys, A., Brozek, J. and Henschel, A. 1950: *The biology of human starvation*. Minneapolis, MN,: University of Minnesota Press.

Ott, L., Young, B., Phillips R. and McClain, C. 1990: Brain injury and nutrition. *Nutrition in Clinical Practice* **5**, 68–73.

Schofield, W.N. 1985: Predicting basal metabolic rate, new standards and review of previous work. *Human Nutrition Clinical Nutrition* **44**, 1–19.

Further reading

Beaufort, Y., Vilae J.P., Annat, G., Delafosse, B., Guillaume, C. and Motin, J. 1987: Energy expenditure in the acute renal failure patient mechanically ventilated. *Intensive Care Medicine* **13**, 404–4.

Daugirdas, J.T. and Todal, S.I. 1994: Nutrition. In *Handbook of dialysis*, 2nd edn. Boston, MA: Little Brown & Co., 377–96.

Elia, M. and Jebb S.A. 1992: Changing concepts of energy requirements of critically ill patients. *Current Medical Literature in Clinical Nutrition* **1**, 35.

Frankenfield, D.C., Wiles, C.E., Bagley, S. and Siegel, J.H. 1994: Relationships between resting and total energy expenditure in injured and septic patients. *Critical Care Medicine* **22**, 1796–804.

Gibson, R.S. 1990: Assessment of protein status. In *Principles of Nutrition Assessment*. New York: Oxford University Press, 313–32.

Kreymann, G., Grosser, S., Buggisch, P., Gottschall, C., Matthael S. and Greten H. 1993: Oxygen consumption and resting metabolic rate in sepsis, sepsis syndrome and septic shock. *Critical Care Medicine* **21**, 1012–19.

McWhirter, J.P. and Pennington C.R. 1994: The incidence and recognition of malnutrition in hospital. *British Medical Journal* **308**, 945–8.

Mattox, T.W. and Teasley-Strausburg, K.M. 1991: Overview of biochemical markers used for nutrition support. *Annals of Pharmacotherapy* **25**, 265–71.

Molina, M.F. and Riella, M.C. 1995: Nutritional support in the patient with renal failure. *Critical Care Clinics* **11**, 685–703.

Parenteral and Enteral Group of the British Dietetic Association 1997: Adult requirements. In: *Pocket guide to clinical nutrition*. Birmingham: British Dietetic Association, 3.1–3.10.

Plauth, M., Merli, M., Kondrup, J., Weimann A., Ferenci P. and Muller, M.J. 1997: Consensus statement. ESPEN guidelines for nutrition in liver disease and transplantation. *Clinical Nutrition* **16**, 43–55.

Appendix 3.1 Estimation of energy and nitrogen requirements for adults

Objectives

- To provide guidelines as to the nutritional requirements for adults requiring enteral or parenteral nutrition

Energy

1. Determine approximate basal metabolic rate (BMR) from Table 3A below.
2. Adjust for stress using nomogram (see Appendix 3.2).
3. Add a combined factor for activity and diet-induced thermogenesis:

Bedbound immobile	+ 10%
Bedbound mobile/sitting	+ 15–20%
Mobile on ward	+ 25%

4. If an increase in energy stores is required, add 400–1000 kcal/day. If a decrease in energy stores is required, reduce energy intake.

When estimating requirements for amputees, it should be noted that although skeletal muscle accounts for about 40% of body weight, it only accounts for approximately 18% of BMR

Table 3A Equations for estimating basal metabolic rate

Females (kcal/day)		Males (kcal/day)	
15–18 years	13.3W* + 690	15–18 years	17.6W + 656
18–30 years	14.8W + 485	18–30 years	15.0W + 690
30–60 years	8.1W + 842	30–60 years	11.4W + 870
> 60 years	9.0W + 656	> 60 years	11.7W + 585

*W = weight expressed in kg.
(Parenteral and Enteral Group of the British Dietetic Association. 1997: Assessment. In *Pocket guide to clinical nutrition.* Birmingham: British Dietetic Association.)

Appendix 3.2 Method for estimating the approximate energy requirements in adult patients receiving artificial nutritional support

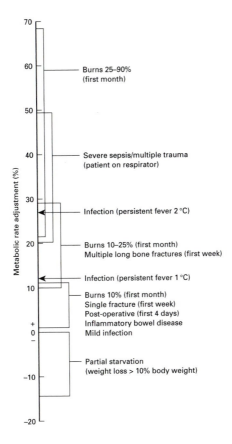

Reprinted with permission. Reproduced from Elia, M. 1990: Artificial nutrition support. *Medicine* **82**, 3394. By kind permission of the Medicine Group (Journals) Ltd.

Appendix 3.3 Electrolyte content of gastrointestinal secretions

Location	Volume (ml)	Na	K	Cl	HCO$_3$
				(mmol/L)	
Gastric juice (fasting)	1500	60	15	90	15
Pancreatic fistula	700	140	5	75	120
Biliary fistula	500	145	5	100	40
Ileostomy	500	115	8	45	30
Diarrhoea	500–1500	120	25	90	45

(Adapted from Pennington, C.R. 1996: Nutritional Requirements. In *Current perspectives on parenteral nutrition in adults.* Bibbenden: British Association for Parenteral and Enteral Nutrition.)

4

The role of the gut

The aims of this chapter are:

- to provide a brief description of the digestive and absorptive role of the gut;
- to outline the gut's immune and barrier function.

Introduction

Recognition of the importance of the gastrointestinal tract and its potential role in the development of multiple organ failure has been increasing over the last 10 years. Prior to this, the gut was thought to be a peripheral organ in the care of the critically ill, of interest only for its potentially damaging role in the development of stress ulceration. Nutrition and the gut were eventually considered once the patient was on the way to recovery.

The gut is now being regarded as an organ that requires support during critical illness in the same way as other primary organs. This is partly due to increased understanding of the role played by the gut in host defence, and the importance of enteral nutrition to immunocompetence.

Three main areas of gut function are important:

- digestion and absorption of nutrients;
- the ability to act as a physical barrier to organisms;
- immune function.

Digestion of nutrients

Digestion is the breakdown by enzymes of compounds in foods into simpler substances that can be assimilated by the body and used in

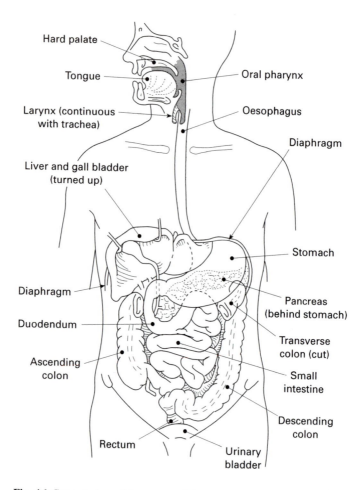

Fig. 4.1 General view of the organs of the digestive tract (reproduced with permission from Ross, J.S. and Wilson, K.J.W. 1973: *Foundations of anatomy and physiology*, 4th edn. Edinburgh: Churchill Livingstone).

metabolic processes. Once food enters the gut, there are three phases of digestion:

1. gut luminal – the secretion of digestive enzymes into the gut lumen;

2. brush border of the gut epithelial cell – further hydrolysis of peptides and disaccharides;
3. cytoplasmic – peptidases reduce peptides to amino acids.

Regulation of mucus and digestive enzyme secretion

Oral and gastric secretions

- These are stimulated by a central response to thinking about food, which affects salivary and gastric secretion – the cephalic phase.
- They are stimulated by a response to the presence of food/chyme in the area of the gut – the gustatory and gastric phase.
- They have a delayed response which continues production even after food has left the area – the gastrointestinal phase.

Pancreatic secretions

- These are stimulated by vagal regulation inducing secretion of high concentrations of enzymes into the ducts. These are flushed through into the small intestine by large quantities of sodium bicarbonate-containing fluid. This fluid is produced in response to secretin release from intestinal mucosa induced by the presence of acidic chyme from the stomach.
- They are stimulated by cholecystokinin release from intestinal mucosa in response to the presence mainly of fats in the small intestine. Cholecystokinin acts on secretory cells in the pancreas to produce large quantities of digestive enzymes.

Liver secretions

The rate of secretion by the liver of bile containing bile salts does not vary, apart from an increase in output of water and sodium bicarbonate in response to secretin release.

Small intestine secretions

These are stimulated by secretion of water, electrolytes, mucus and digestive enzymes, this being regulated by local nervous reflexes (i.e. local distension of the gastrointestinal tract).

There may also be a hormonal mechanism, but as yet this has not been identified.

Table 4.1 Digestion of nutrients

	Mouth		Stomach		Duodenum/jejunum	
	Digested by the enzymes	Absorbed	Digested by the enzymes	Absorbed	Digested by the enzymes	Absorbed
Proteins	–	No	Pepsin	No	Trypsin, chymotrypsin elastase, carboxy-peptidases	Yes
Carbohydrates	Salivary amalyse	No		Yes (glucose only)	Amylase, maltase, lactase, sucrase	Yes
Fats	Lingual lipase	No	Hydrochloric acid, gastric lipase	No	Bile salts (from gall bladder) cholesterol esterase, lipase	Yes

Luminal digestive enzymes (apart from salivary amylase, lingual and gastric lipase and pepsin) are secreted by the pancreas and activated by the environment of the small intestine. Brush-border enzymes are also secreted in the epithelial cells of the small intestine. The small intestine is therefore the most important site for digestion and absorption, and intestinal function is preserved here even when there is evidence of dysfunction in other parts of the gut.

Factors affecting digestion in the critically ill

- Brush-border enzymes secreted by the epithelial cells are induced by the presence of luminal nutrients, and enzyme activity is decreased when these are absent, e.g. when patients are starved or receiving parenteral nutrition (PN).
- Malnutrition leads to digestive enzyme deficiencies, particularly those enzymes secreted by luminal cells (i.e. the brush-border membrane).
- Critically ill patients may develop disaccharidase deficiency (lactase, sucrase, maltase). Therefore lactose-free enteral feeding products are commonly used.
- Pancreatic insufficiency and loss of brush-border enzymes can occur following infection, gut atrophy and mucosal damage. Protein digestion can be limited as a result.
- Diminished mucus secretion and atrophy of enterocytes may occur in critical illness.

Many of these factors will apply to the critically ill patient, e.g. previous malnutrition, periods of starvation, infection, etc. It is important that enteral nutrition is seen as a priority, and that the patient's response is monitored to ensure that early evidence of dysfunction is identified.

Absorption of nutrients

Absorption takes place primarily in the small intestine, which is one of the most resilient sections of the gut. It remains motile and able to

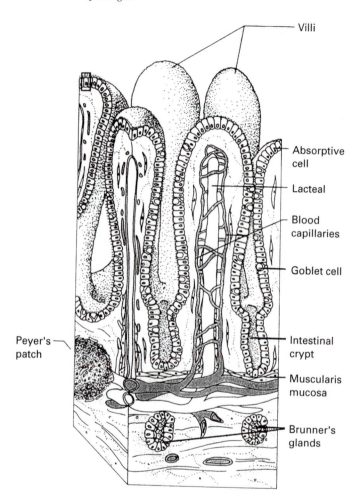

Fig. 4.2 Cross-section of the intestinal villus with blood supply.

absorb nutrients even when the stomach and colon are virtually atonic. There is a number of feedback mechanisms (see Box 4.1) which ensure that movement of nutrients through the gut is as smooth as possible. Luminal nutrients are vital for maintaining efficient absorption and, where possible, enteral nutrition should always continue.

Box 4.1 Factors affecting movement of nutrients through the gut

1. Gastric to duodenal delivery of nutrients – antral peristalsis and fundal tone are reduced by the arrival of nutrients and hyperosmolar solutions in the duodenum, maintaining a fairly constant delivery of 1–2 kcal/min.
2. Malabsorbed nutrients (particularly fat) are detected by sensors in the ileum which exert a further inhibitory effect on gastric emptying and duodenal and jejunal motility.
3. Addition of fibre may reduce absorption of glucose, which then has an inhibitory effect on total transit time (mouth to caecum).

Effective absorption is dependent on adequate mixing of food-stuff. This has two functions:

- to allow breakdown of food into chyme;
- to allow presentation of digestible nutrients to the brush-border membrane.

Transit of gut contents is designed to occur at a continuous, non-pulsatile rate to aid absorption, and is probably improved by the slow continuous delivery of enteral feeds, especially into the duodenum. However, Raimundo *et al.* (1988, 1989) and Dive *et al.*, (1994) have shown that continuous delivery of enteral feed into the stomach is associated with increased secretion of fluid into the colon and abnormal continuation of migrating motor complexes. These highly propulsive contractions, in combination with increased fluid in the colon, can be associated with diarrhoea. It may therefore be best to feed continually post-pylorus rather than intragastrically, but this has yet to be resolved.

Factors affecting absorption in the critically ill

These include:

- intestinal villous atrophy which results in a reduction in the surface area available for absorption – this can be caused by protein malnutrition, lack of enteral feeding and ischaemia;
- digestive enzyme deficiency related to malnutrition;
- an inappropriately high rate of intestinal transit – this may be a feature of organ dysfunction, or it can be caused by drugs used in

critically ill patients, such as inotropes, antibiotics (erythromycin) and gut motility stimulants such as metaclopromide or cisapride;

- delayed gastric emptying is common in the critically ill (see Factors Affecting Gastric Emptying, Table 4.2), and this may decrease the rate of protein assimilation by limiting the flow of nutrients to the absorptive surface;
- secretion of gastric acid may be reduced in the critically ill (Higgins *et al.*, 1994);
- bacterial overgrowth following bowel stasis can result in bacterial modification of bile acids and deactivation of mucosal digestive enzymes;
- pseudomembranous colitis may develop as a side-effect of antibiotic usage.

Table 4.2 Factors affecting gastric emptying

Factors which reduce emptying	Factors which increase emptying
Hyperosmolality of feed	Motility-stimulating drugs, e.g.
High fat content	erythromycin, cisapride, domperidone
High fibre content	Fluid contents
Critical illness	
Acidic duodenal pH	
Motility-depressant drugs, e.g. opiates, sedatives	

The splanchnic circulation

The splanchnic circulation (Fig. 4.3) supplies the stomach (including the lower portion of the oesophagus), the small and large bowel, the liver, the gall-bladder, the pancreas and the spleen. It has a high blood flow (approximately 30 per cent of cardiac output in the healthy individual) and a large reservoir function. Splanchnic vasoconstriction can provide up to 70 per cent of the venous reservoir available as a response to hypovolaemia. The splanchnic organs are therefore particularly vulnerable during hypovolaemia and decreased cardiac output to reduction and redistribution of blood flow. The epithelial cells of the gastrointestinal tract are also among the fastest proliferating in the body, with high normal oxygen requirements.

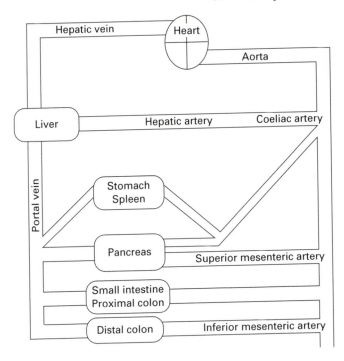

Fig. 4.3 The splanchnic circulation – major blood vessels and organs.

These are compromised during prolonged periods of vasoconstriction, leading to tissue hypoxia and ultimately necrosis.

Gut immune function

The gut lumen is in constant contact with potentially toxic substances such as micro-organisms, endotoxins, etc. It requires an enormously complex but highly effective system of defence to prevent penetration by these substances into the vulnerable underlying tissues and systemic circulation (Fig. 4.4).

The key gut immune functions are:

- the generation of secretory IgA antibody;
- local cellular immunity;

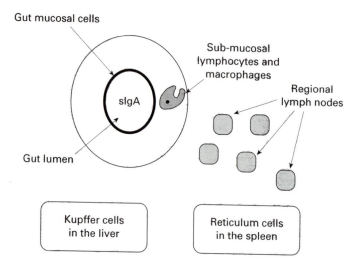

Fig. 4.4 Gut immune function.

- down-regulation of systemic immunity to antigens presented through the gut.

These functions are primarily protective against continuous exposure to ingested organisms in the gut lumen. They are dependent on nutrients and gut luminal contents to function effectively.

Bacterial translocation

The penetration of the protective barrier of the gut by organisms/endotoxins is known as bacterial translocation.

Bacterial translocation occurs in two ways:

- invasion of the intestinal mucosa by specific enteric pathogens, e.g. *Salmonella, Listeria, Campylobacter*. This is associated with either destruction of normal epithelium or a previously injured, inflamed or abnormal area of epithelium;
- migration of indigenous bacterial species across the intestinal epithelium.

It is clear that bacterial translocation *per se* can occur in the critically ill (Lipman, 1995). However, there is little evidence that it is associated with septic morbidity.

Physiological gut defence mechanisms

The gut has its own less specialized lymphoid areas which behave to some extent as a separate lymphatic circuit. The highly concentrated collection of lymph nodules and Peyer's patches found throughout the gut is known collectively as the gut-associated lymphoid tissue (GALT). There are as many lymphocytes in 2 metres of the gut as in the whole of the marrow, spleen and lymph nodes (Playfair, 1996).

The following mechanisms also work in tandem to ensure protection from invading organisms within the gut lumen:

- bactericidal pH in gastric acid;
- production and secretion of mucus (to protect enterocytes from luminal contents and to prevent adherence of organisms to the mucosa);
- production of secretory immunoglobulin A (sIgA) by Peyer's patches (sIgA prevents adherence of bacteria to the mucosal cells);
- a physical barrier from the gut mucosa with tight junctions between epithelial cells;
- high numbers of lymphocytes and macrophages in the intestinal walls;
- dense mesenteric lymph nodes;
- the presence of organ-specific macrophages (Kupffer cells) in the liver and reticulo-endothelial cells in the spleen to filter, trap and phagocytose organisms in the hepatic portal circulation;
- enteric nervous system sensitization to antigens involving local vasodilation, secretion of large amounts of water, electrolytes and mucoproteins, and increased motility.

These mechanisms are normally sufficient to limit any bacterial/endotoxin challenge made in the absence of systemic illness.

Factors which may contribute to failure of immune function in the gut

These include the following:

- altered permeability or loss of integrity of the mucosa as a result of hypovolaemic ischaemia, sepsis or endotoxaemia. These are compounded by starvation or protein malnutrition and possibly by the use of parenteral rather than enteral nutrition;

- decreased host defence mechanisms such as immunosuppression related to sepsis, steroid use, chemotherapy, etc;
- increased bacterial numbers within the intestine secondary to overgrowth as a result of antibiotic treatment, or to intestinal stasis.

Both starvation and protein malnutrition have been shown to impair host immune defences, disrupt the balance of the normal gut flora and produce gut mucosal atrophy.

Factors affecting gut mucosal permeability

These include:

- hypoperfusion related to hypovolaemia;
- ischaemia related to hypoxaemia and hypoperfusion;
- malnutrition and nutrition modes and novel substrates;
- Sepsis and endotoxins.

Factors which may contribute to improved immune function in the gut

These include:

- early enteral feeding;
- content of enteral feeds;
- support of gastrointestinal blood flow.

Early enteral feeding

Research suggests that early enteral feeding (i.e. within 6 h of insult) can modify the hormonal response to stress (Mochizuki *et al.*, 1984; Fong *et al.*, 1989), improve wound healing (Delaney *et al.*, 1989; Zaloga *et al.*, 1992) and possibly decrease the incidence of bowel obstruction (Schroeder *et al.*, 1991).

Content of enteral feeds

Some nutrients themselves may also have immunomodulatory properties (see Chapters 2 and 5). Actions include stimulating growth hormone, supporting enterocyte and lymphocyte function, altering prostaglandin release in response to inflammation, and acting as a colonocyte fuel source. Therefore there may well be a role for the so-called immunonutrient agents, e.g. omega-3/6 fatty acids, arginine.

Nutrients that are thought to affect immune function include:

- arginine;
- glutamine;
- omega-3/6 fatty acids;
- nucleotides.

Support of improved gastrointestinal blood flow

Constriction of the splanchnic bed is the body's response to conditions involving hypovolaemia or hypotension. This response is effective when it is short term, but becomes rapidly degenerative when it is continued until gut tissue hypoxia and cell death occur. Mucosal hypoxia is evident even with a modest decrease in gut perfusion, and necrosis of villi occurs within minutes (Fiddian-Green, 1988). Further disruption of the mucosal barrier is aided by the presence of acid, bile, digestive enzymes or bacteria and bacterial products in the lumen. Intestinal barrier disruption increases vulnerability to intraluminal organisms, which may lead to bacteraemia or sepsis.

Immune enhancement by enteral feeding

- Lymphocyte, neutrophil and gut-associated immune function are better preserved than in parenterally fed subjects (Zaloga, 1994).
- Enteral presentation of foodstuffs is an absolute requirement for maintenance of gut metabolic and immune function (Alverdy *et al.*, 1985).
- Production of sIgA is enhanced by enteral nutrients (Alverdy *et al.*, 1985).
- Attenuation of the catabolic response is seen in subjects fed immediately post-insult (Mochizuki *et al.*, 1984; Fong *et al.*, 1989).
- Significantly fewer infectious complications (e.g. pneumonia, abscesses, empyema) are seen in trauma patients (Kudsk *et al.*, 1992; Kudsk, 1994; Moore *et al.*, 1995).

The evidence suggests that it is beneficial to maintain enteral nutrition for as long as possible in the critically ill patient in order to sustain the immunological defence role of the gut.

References

Alverdy, J., Chi, H.S. and Sheldon, G.F. 1985: The effect of parenteral nutrition on gastrointestinal immunity. *Annals of Surgery* **202**, 681–4.

Delaney, H.M., Demetriou, A.A., Teh, E. and Levenson, S.M. 1989: Effect of early postoperative nutritional support on skin wound and colon anastomosis healing. *Journal of Parenteral and Enteral Nutrition* **14**, 357–61.

Dive, A., Miesse, C., Jamart, J., Evrard, P., Gonzalez, M. and Installe, E.T. 1994: Duodenal motor response to continuous enteral feeding is impaired in mechanically ventilated critically ill patients. *Clinical Nutrition* **13**, 302–6.

Fiddian-Green, R.G. 1988: Splanchnic ischaemia and multiple organ failure in the critically ill. *Annals of the Royal College of Surgeons of England* **70**, 128–34.

Fong, Y., Marano, M.A., Barber, A. *et al.*, 1989: Total parenteral nutrition and bowel rest modify the metabolic response to endotoxin in humans. *Annals of Surgery* **210**, 449–56.

Higgins, D.J., Mythen, M.G. and Webb, A.R. 1994: Low intramucosal pH is associated with failure to acidify the gastric lumen in response to pentagastrin. *Intensive Care Medicine* **20**, 105–8.

Kudsk, K.A. 1994: Gut mucosal nutritional support – enteral nutrition as primary therapy after multiple system trauma. *Gut* Suppl. **1**, S52–S54.

Kudsk, K.A., Croce, M.A., Fabian, T.C. *et al.*, 1992: Enteral versus parenteral feeding. *Annals of Surgery* **215**, 503–11.

Lipman, T.O. 1995: Bacterial translocation and enteral nutrition in humans: an outsider looks in. *Journal of Parenteral and Enteral Nutrition* **19**, 156–65.

Mochizuki, H., Trocki, O., Dominioni, L. *et al.*, 1984: Mechanism of prevention of postburn hypermetabolism and catabolism by early enteral feeding. *Annals of Surgery* **200**, 297–310.

Moore, F.A., Moore, E.E. and Haenel, J.B. 1995: Clinical benefits of early post-injury feeding. *Clinical Intensive Care* **6**, 21–7.

Playfair, J.M.L. 1996: *Immunology at a glance*, 6th Edn. Oxford: Blackwell Science.

Raimundo, A.H., Rogers, J., Grimble, G.K., Cahill, E. and Silk, D.B.A. 1988: Colonic inflow and small bowel motility during intraduodenal enteral nutrition. *Gut* **29**, 1469–70 (abstract).

Raimundo, A.H., Rogers, J., Spiller, R.C., Grimble, G.K. and Silk, D.B.A. 1989: Effect of continuous intraduodenal enteral feeding on human colonic in-flow volumes and small bowel motility. *Gastroenterology* **404**, 96 (abstract).

Schroeder, D., Gillanders, L., Mahr, K. and Hill, G.L. 1991: Effects of immediate postoperative enteral nutrition on body composition, muscle function, and wound healing. *Journal of Parenteral and Enteral Nutrition* **15**, 376–83.

Zaloga, G.P. 1994: *Nutrition in critical care*. Philadelphia, PA: Mosby.

Zaloga, G.P., Bortenschlager, L., Black, K.W. and Prielipp, R. 1992: Immediate postoperative enteral feeding decreases weight loss and improves wound healing after abdominal surgery in rats. *Critical Care Medicine* **20**, 115–18.

Further reading

Johnson, L.R. 1997: *Gastrointestinal physiology*. St Louis, MO: Mosby – Year Book Inc.

Schiller, L.R. 1994: Peristalsis. *Scientific American* **Nov/Dec**, 38–47.

Schlichtig, R. and Ayres, S.M. 1988: Nutritional support of the critically ill. Chicago, IL: Year Book Medical Publishers.

5

Content of enteral feeds

The aims of this chapter are:

- to describe the range of feeds available;
- to explain the rationale for their use.

There is a wide variety of feeds available, a number of which have specific applications in the critically ill which will be described below.

As discussed in Chapter 3, for all patients the following factors need to be taken into consideration before selecting the correct formula:

- nutritional requirements of the individual;
- nutritional status *prior to* ICU admission, e.g. cachexia, anorexia, periods of NBM on ward, alcoholism, COAD and CCF, all of which will decrease nutritional intake over time;
- diagnosis;
- the refeeding syndrome, which is characterized by severe hypo-phosphataemia and other metabolic complications seen in mal-nourished patients receiving concentrated calories after a period of starvation;
- type of ventilatory support;
- other i.v. fluids/drugs being administered, e.g. dextrose saline, electrolytes, propofol.

Content of feeds

In general most feeds contain protein, carbohydrate, fat, electrolytes, trace elements, minerals, vitamins and water, and are nutritionally complete.

The proteins may be in the form of intact protein (casein) or peptides, or as amino acids. Similarly, the carbohydrate may be provided as complex starches (polysaccharides), glucose polymers (cornstarch), or as simple monosaccharides (glucose).

Fat is usually in the form of long-chain triglycerides, although there are some feeds in which MCTs predominate.

In general, the more hydrolysed (predigested) the feed, the higher the osmolality and the less enzyme activity is required for digestion. Absorption will still require some functional capacity of the small bowel. The osmolality of a given feed should not affect tolerance provided that introduction to the full-strength feed is managed in a time-controlled fashion.

Allison (1986) has pointed out the importance of osmol administered per unit time rather than per unit volume.

Osmolality and *osmolarity* are both terms referring to the molar concentration of a solute in a solution.

- Osmolality is the number of osmotically active particles added to a kilogram of water.
- Osmolarity is the number of osmotically active particles made up to 1 litre of solution in water.

The average osmolality of a standard feed is 280–300 mosmol/kg H_2O.

Feeds are available in different forms, e.g. liquid and powder, and in a number of formats, e.g. can, bottle, ready to hang, etc.

The ready-to-hang presentation is ideal for use in the ICU as it is available in 500-mL, or 1-L or 1500-mL volumes and does not require decanting before administration. This has obvious microbiological advantages in that it reduces handling of the giving set and reservoir and subsequent microbial contamination (Anderton, 1993).

Enteral feeds fall into four main categories and will be discussed in the following order:

- standard polymeric formulae;
- modified mineral/electrolyte formulae;
- elemental/semi-elemental formulae;
- specialist feeds.

Standard polymeric formulae

Profile

100 mL provide 100 kcal of energy
  ~ 4 g of protein
  ~ 4 mmol of sodium
  ~ 4 mmol of potassium
(see Appendix 5.1).

Polymeric feeds contain nutrients in their intact form, i.e. as proteins, fats and carbohydrates. They are all lactose- and gluten free and are generally hyperosmolar. Some feeds are isotonic, i.e. they have the same osmolality as plasma (150 mosmol/L) and some are pre-diluted.

Rationale for use

In a typical 2000-mL feed, 2000 kcal of energy and approximately 70 g of protein would be provided to meet 'average' nutritional requirements. These feeds may be used for patients with pre-existing malnutrition or those who are at risk of malnutrition. They are also indicated for patients with malignant disease and minor burns (< 10 per cent of total body surface area). This is the usual feed for supporting the critically ill patient.

Clinical evidence

Iso-osmolar feeds/pre-diluted feeds

These are advocated for use as starter regimens to decrease gut intolerance in patients who are likely to be susceptible, or to decrease diarrhoea. However, there is no evidence to suggest that these feeds confer any benefit in the critically ill.

This is because the rate of gastric emptying during enteral feeding is controlled by the energy content and *not* by the osmolality of the diet. Keohane *et al.* (1984) demonstrated that there was no benefit conferred by the use of starter regimens for enterally fed patients. *In-vivo* human perfusion studies (Raimundo *et al.*, 1992) have shown that the absorptive capacity of the colon is capable of handling feed volumes should post-pyloric feeding be considered.

Pre-diluted feeds, e.g. Pre-Nutrison (Nutricia) and Introlite (Ross) are consequently not advocated in the ICU setting, where starter regimens have little if any advantage, particularly when they delay the attainment of nutritional targets.

Energy-dense feeds

Profile

100 mL provide ~ 150–200 kcal of energy
  ~ 5–8 g of protein
  ~ 4–5 mmol of sodium
  ~ 4–5 mmol of potassium
(see Appendix 5.2).

Rationale for use

These are advocated for patients with increased energy and protein requirements, e.g. those with burns, multiple trauma, etc., who may not tolerate the high volumes of standard feed required. Patients requiring a fluid-restricted regimen or overnight feeding may also benefit from the use of these feeds.

Fibre-enriched feeds

Profile

These feeds have a protein and energy profile similar to that of standard polymeric feeds, apart from the fact that they are supplemented with dietary fibre (see Appendix 5.3).

Rationale for use

These are advocated to aid normal bowel function.

Clinical evidence

Bowling (1995) proposed that disordered colonic function was a cause of enteral feed-related diarrhoea.

Short-chain fatty acids (SCFA), i.e. proprionic, acetic and butyric acids, are produced as a result of fermentation of soluble fibre provided in the enteral feed. These acids act as powerful stimulants to water and sodium absorption in the colon, and are believed to be used preferentially as a fuel by colonocytes. Feeds containing soluble fibre as soy polysaccharides may be of benefit in decreasing diarrhoea. Some fibre-containing feeds contain insoluble fibre which will not alter SCFA concentrations and will only increase stool bulk.

Modified mineral/electrolyte feeds

Low-sodium feeds

Rationale for use

These are advocated for patients requiring a sodium-restricted feed, e.g. in cardiac, renal and liver failure or in acute head injury where ICP is elevated. Low sodium feeds should only be used if there is significant hypernatraemia, i.e. > 150 mmol/L. A 24-h urinary sodium or a single measurement of urinary sodium should be obtained to ensure that the problem is not caused by dehydration.

Nutrison low sodium (Nutricia) is the only low-sodium feed available on the UK market. It is supplied in a 500-mL bottle.

Profile

100 mL provide   100 kcal of energy
4 g of protein
1.1 mmol of sodium
3.5 mmol of potassium.

Low-protein/low-mineral feeds

Rationale for use

These are advocated for patients requiring restricted fluid, protein and mineral intake, e.g. in cases of hepatic encephalopathy, and end-stage renal failure where renal replacement therapy is not available or is not indicated.

Profile

1. Nutrison low-protein/low-minerals (Nutricia), supplied in a 500-mL bottle.

   100 mL provide 200 kcal of energy
   4 g of protein
   4.3 mmol of sodium
   3.8 mmol of potassium.

2. Suplena (Ross), supplied in a 237-mL can.

   100 mL provide 201 kcal of energy
   3 g of protein
   3.48 mmol of sodium
   2.87 mmol of potassium.

3. Clinifeed iso (Nestlé Clinical), supplied in a 375-mL can.

   100 mL provide 100 kcal of energy
   2.8 g of protein
   1.5 mmol of sodium
   3.8 mmol of potassium.

High-energy/low-electrolyte feeds

Rationale for use

These are advocated for patients on haemodialysis, especially if continuous, where amino acid losses are large (Bellomo *et al.*, 1991).

Profile

1. Nepro (Ross), supplied in a 237-mL can.

   100 mL provide 200 kcal of energy
   7.0 g of protein
   3.48 mmol of sodium
   2.69 mmol of potassium.

2. Nutrison concentrated LE (Nutricia), supplied in a 500-mL bottle.

   100 mL provide 200 kcal of energy
   7.5 g of protein
   4.3 mmol of sodium
   3.8 mmol of potassium.

Semi-elemental/elemental feeds

Semi-elemental feeds

Profile

A wide variety of feeds fall into this category, and their profiles are variable depending on their indications for use. In general, however, the protein is present in the feed as peptides, the fat as medium-chain triglycerides and the carbohydrate as maltodextrins, which are more readily absorbed by the gut and therefore may confer some benefit in conditions such as malabsorption, inflammatory bowel disease and Crohn's disease.

Such feeds are lactose and gluten free and are often also fructose, sucrose and milk-protein free (see Appendix 5.4).

Elemental feeds

Profile

All nutrients are present in elemental form, i.e. carbohydrates are present as simple sugars (monosaccharides), proteins as amino acids and fats as fatty acids.

Rationale for use

These are advocated in severe malabsorption, bowel fistulae, short bowel syndrome, irritable bowel syndrome and Crohn's disease.

Feeds

1. Elemental O28 (SHS).
2. Elemental O28 Extra (SHS) – increased nitrogen, fat (35 per cent MCT) and energy content compared with Elemental O28, and supplemented with glutamine and arginine.
3. Emsogen (SHS) – supplemented with glutamine and arginine and 83 per cent MCT. Advocated for patients with severe malabsorption, e.g. cystic fibrosis, HIV infection, where long-chain triglycerides (LCTs) are poorly tolerated.

Specialist feeds for the critically ill

Profile 1

Supplemented with glutamine and/or arginine, nucleotides, omega-3 fatty acids and antioxidants.

Glutamine

Rationale for use

Glutamine is an amino acid which appears to become conditionally essential after major trauma/stress. Under normal circumstances the body is able to synthesize glutamine, normal intake being 4–5 g daily.

However, in illness, requirements increase markedly and if adequate glutamine is not provided, net catabolism of skeletal muscle can occur to supply the requirements of glutamine-dependent tissues. Current enteral feeds appear to contain insufficient glutamine under such conditions (see Chapter 2 for details of the properties of glutamine).

Clinical evidence

Few studies have been published on the efficacy of glutamine-supplemented enteral nutrition in the critically ill. However, Griffiths *et al.* (1997) performed a randomized double-blind trial in 156 critically ill patients (Apache score > 11).

These patients were randomized to receive either glutamine-supplemented enteral feeds or standard enteral feeds. If they were unable to tolerate enteral feeds, they received glutamine-supplemented PN or standard PN. Outcome measures were morbidity and cost. In the glutamine-supplemented PN group, the survival rate was 57 per cent, compared with 33 per cent in the control group at 6 months. There was a 50 per cent reduction in cost. There was no significant difference in mortality between the enterally and parenterally fed groups. However, the glutamine-supplemented PN group had a reduced hospital stay and a 30 per cent reduction in hospital costs.

Glutamine-supplemented formulae

1. AlitraQ (Ross), supplied in powder form in a 76-g sachet.
   Provides 18 g of glutamine per 2000 kcal.
2. Protina G (Oxford Nutrition), supplied in a 107-g bottle.
   Provides 21.6 g of glutamine per 2000 kcal.

Arginine

Rationale for use

Arginine is an essential amino acid for growth, and it may become essential, like glutamine, in the catabolic state. Normal intakes of arginine in the average Western diet are 5.4 g L-arginine daily.

It is postulated that, in the critically ill, supplementation is essential to support the immune response.

Clinical evidence

Arginine-supplemented formulae improve nitrogen balance and wound healing, stimulate the T-cell response and reduce infections (see Chapter 2 for details of the properties of arginine).

Nucleotides

Dietary RNA may be necessary to maintain the immune response in the critically ill. However, in a recent review by Heyland *et al.* (1995) it was concluded that there was as yet little evidence to support the use of RNA supplementation in the prevention of infectious complications in the critically ill.

Omega-3 fatty acids

It is suggested that the ratio of omega-3 fatty acids to omega-6 fatty acids can alter the types of eicosanoids produced by cells as part of the immune response (see Chapter 2 for details of the properties of omega-3 fatty acids).

Clinical evidence

To date, most of the research has been done in animals, and these studies have not all shown benefits.

Omega-3 fatty acid supplementation blocks production of the prostaglandin PG_2. The actual role of this prostaglandin in the immune response is not clearly defined, and it may in fact have an advantageous immune effect in the early stages of sepsis or trauma, by suppressing the release of TNF.

Omega-3 fatty acids also reduce thromboxane activity. Thromboxane is an eicosanoid which plays an important role in the maintenance of vascular tone, and in platelet aggregation.

Another cause for concern is that diets high in PUFAs can lead to the production of free radicals and lipid peroxides which can cause cellular and tissue damage.

Antioxidants

These include the vitamins, beta-carotene, vitamins C and E and also trace elements, e.g. selenium. These substances can influence the oxidative modification of lipoproteins in the arterial wall, and can prevent the harmful effects of the free radical chain reactions.

To date there have been no studies to support the supplementation of antioxidants in the critically ill.

In the UK there are no feeds available supplemented *solely* with arginine, RNA, omega-3 fatty acids or antioxidants. However, there are feeds which are supplemented with combinations of these nutrients, and these will be discussed below.

1. Impact (Novartis Nutrition UK Ltd) – supplemented with RNA, glutamine and arginine.
2. Perative (Ross) – supplemented with arginine and omega-3 fatty acids.

Clinical evidence

The feed impact has been evaluated in the critically ill with varying degrees of success.

Cerra *et al.* (1991) randomized 20 critically ill trauma patients to Impact or a standard feed. They demonstrated greater immune cell proliferation *in vitro*, but there were no differences in infections or mortality. The sample size was too small to determine the difference in infectious morbidity or mortality rates.

A larger study by Bower *et al.* (1995) of 326 critically ill patients failed to demonstrate an overall reduction in infection rates. However, in the septic group there was a 40 per cent reduction in hospital stay and a 60 per cent lower incidence of nosocomial pneumonia.

Profile 2

High-fat low-carbohydrate feed.

Rationale for use

This is advocated to reduce CO_2 production in the ventilated patient. This feed contains 55 per cent fat and 31.5 per cent carbohydrate, and therefore has a lower RQ than a standard feed containing around 28 per cent fat and 55 per cent carbohydrate (note that the RQ for fat is 0.7 and the RQ for carbohydrate is 1.0).

Pulmocare (Abbott Labs)

100 mL provide 150 kcal of energy
6.25 g of protein
5.65 mmol of sodium
4.46 mmol of potassium.

Case studies

Case study 1

A 54-year-old man (weighing 40 kg) is admitted to hospital with ascites, jaundice, low-grade pyrexia, a reported weight loss of 4 kg in the last month due to loss of appetite, and anaemia and thrombocytopenia.

- Previous medical history – alcoholic liver disease.
- History of alcohol abuse (2 bottles of wine daily). Attends a centre for alcohol abuse.
- The patient is transferred to the ICU with increasing respiratory dependency, borderline renal failure, deranged clotting and possible pulmonary oedema.
- A diagnosis of encephalopathy (Grade II) and possible aspiration pneumonia is made.

- The patient is intubated and ventilated due to increasing respiratory distress. Enteral feeding is commenced. Biochemistry is as follows:

urea	21.7 mmol/L
sodium	123 mmol/L
potassium	4.5 mmol/L
creatinine	137 μmol/L
bilirubin	260 μmol/L
ALP	432 IU/L
AST	64 IU/L
calcium	2.07 mmol/L
phosphate	0.97 mmol/L
albumin	30 g/L.

1. What are this patient's requirements?
2. Which feed would you choose to meet these requirements?

Case study 2

A 68-year-old woman (weighing 65 kg) is transferred to the ICU with respiratory failure, pulmonary haemorrhage, vasculitis and deteriorating renal function.

- Previous medical history – splenectomy, hyperthyroidism, previous deep venous thrombosis (DVT).
- On admission the patient is intubated and ventilated, and enteral feeding commences on a standard polymeric feed.
- She is started on renal dopamine to improve urine output, but eventually requires continuous haemofiltration.
- At this stage she is tolerating 1800 mL of a standard polymeric feed.
- She is referred to the renal team as weaning off the ventilator progresses, and they indicate that she is ready for intermittent dialysis.
- Her biochemistry at this stage is as follows:

urea	17.2 mmol/L
sodium	130 mmol/L
potassium	4.1 mmol/L

creatinine	195 μmol/L
calcium	2.02 mmol/L
phosphate	1.14 mmol/L
ALP	426 IU/L
AST	31 IU/L
magnesium	1.05 mmol/L
albumin	16 g/L.

1. What factors in her current feeding regimen need to be taken into consideration when she goes on to intermittent dialysis?

References

Allison, S.P. 1986: How I feed patients enterally. *Proceedings of the Nutrition Society* **45**, 163–9.

Anderton, A. 1993: Bacterial contamination of enteral feeds and feeding systems. *Clinical Nutrition* **12**, 16–33.

Bellomo, R., Martin, H., Parkin, G., Love, J., Kearley, Y. and Boyce, N. 1991: Continuous arteriovenous haemodiafiltration in the critically ill; influence on major nutrient balances. *Intensive Care Medicine* **17**, 399–402.

Bower, R.H., Lavin, P.T. and LiCari, J.J. 1995: A modified enteral formula reduces hospital length of stay in patients in intensive care units. *Critical Care Medicine* **23**, 436–49.

Bowling, T.E. 1995: Enteral feeding-related diarrhoea: proposed causes and possible solutions. *Proceedings of the Nutrition Society* **54**, 579–90.

Cerra, F.B., Lehmann, S., Konstantinides, N. *et al.* 1991: Improvement in immune function in ICU patients by enteral nutrition supplemented with arginine, RNA and Menhaden oil is independent of nitrogen balance. *Nutrition* **7** 193–9.

Griffiths, R.D., Jones, C. and Palmer, T.E.A. 1997: Six-month outcome of critically ill patients given glutamine-supplemented parenteral nutrition. *Nutrition* **13**, 2–9.

Heyland, D.K., Cook, D.J. and Guyatt, G.H. 1995: Does the formulation of enteral feeding products influence the infectious morbidity and mortality rates in the critically ill patient? *Critical Care Medicine* **22**, 1192–202.

Raimundo, A.H., Jameson, J.S., Rogers, J. and Silk, D.B.A. 1992: The effect of enteral nutrition on distal colonic motility. *Gastroenterology* **102**, 573 (abstract).

Further reading

Bowling, T.E., Raimundo, A.H., Grimble, G.K. and Silk, D.B.A. 1993: Reversal by short-chain fatty acids of colonic fluid secretion induced by enteral feeding. *Lancet* **342**, 1266–8.

Bowling, T.E., Raimundo, A.H. and Silk, D.B.A. 1993: The effect of enteral feeding on colonic water absorption in man. *Gastroenterology* **104**, 610 (abstract).

Daly, J.M, Reynolds, M.B., Thom, A. *et al.* 1998: Immune and metabolic effects of arginine in the surgical patient. *Annals of Surgery* **208**, 512–23.

Kapadia, S.A., Raimundo, A.H., and Silk, D.B.A. 1991: Intestinal function in normal volunteers consuming normal diet and polymeric enteral diet with and without added soy-polysaccharide. *Clinical Nutrition* **10** (Suppl. 2), 42–5.

Keohane, P.P., Attill, H., Love, M., Frost, P. and Silk, D.B.A. 1984: Relation between osmolality and gastrointestinal side-effects in enteral nutrition. *British Medical Journal* **288**, 678–80.

Kinsella, J.E. 1990: Dietary polyunsaturated fatty acids and eicosanoids: potential effects on the modulation of inflammatory and immune cells. An overview. *Nutrition* **6**, 24–44.

Kirk, S.J. and Barbul, A. 1990: Role of arginine in trauma, sepsis and immunity. *Journal of Parenteral and Enteral Nutrition* **14**, 226S–229S.

Peck, M.D. 1994: Omega-3 polyunsaturated fatty acids: benefits of harm during sepsis. *New Horizons* **2**, 230–36.

Souba, W.W. 1990: Glutamine nutrition: theoretical considerations and therapeutic impact. *Journal of Parenteral and Enteral Nutrition* **14**, 237S–243S.

Appendix 5.1 Standard polymeric feeds: composition and manufacturer

Feed	Company	Presentation
Ensure	Ross	250-mL can/500-mL bottle
Osmolite	Ross	1/1.5-L RTH/500-mL bottle/250-mL can
Nutrison	Nutricia	1-L RTH/500-mL bottle
Fresubin	Fresenius	500-mL bottle/500-mL Easy Bag
Clinifeed 1.0	Nestlé Clinical	375-mL can/500-mL/1-L Dripac-flex
Nutrison soya*	Nutricia	1-L RTH/500-mL bottle

*indicated for vegans.

Appendix 5.2 Energy dense feeds: composition and manufacturer

Feed	Company	Energy (kcal/mL)	Presentation
Ensure plus	Ross	1.5	500-mL bottle/1-L RTH
Two Cal HN	Ross	2.0	237-mL can
Nutrison energy	Nutricia	1.5	500-mL bottle/1-L RTH
Entera	Fresenius	1.5	500-mL bottle/500-mL Easy Bag
Clinifeed 1.5	Nestlé Clinical	1.5	500-mL/1-L Dripac-flex

Appendix 5.3 Fibre-enriched feeds: composition and manufacturer

Feed	Company	Fibre (g/100 mL)	Presentation
Enrich	Ross	1.4	250-mL can
Jevity*	Ross	1.4	500-mL bottle/1-L or 1.5-L RTH
Fresubin isofibre*	Fresenius	1.5	500-mL bottle/500-mL or 1-L Easy Bag
Nutrison fibre*	Nutricia	1.5	500-mL bottle spike and hang/1-L RTH
Clinifeed fibre (contains: 50% soluble fibre)	Nestlé Clinical	1.5	500-mL/1-L Dripac-flex

RTH/Easy Bag/DRIPAC-flex are ready-to-hang presentations. *Contains soluble fibre.

Appendix 5.4 Modified mineral/electrolyte feeds: composition and manufacturer

Feed	Company	Content	Presentation
Pepti-2000 LF	Nutricia	15–20% AAs 75–80% peptides 50% MCT	500-mL bottle/1-L RTH/126-g powder
Liquisorbon MCT	Nutricia	70% MCT	500-mL bottle
Peptide 2+	SHS	83% MCT	400-g powder
Pepatamen	Nestlé Clinical	99% peptides 70% MCT	375-mL can
Perative	Ross	15% AAs 20% peptides 40% MCT	237-mL can/1-L RTH
Survimed OPD	Fresenius	15% AAs 50% peptides 50% MCT	500-mL bottle/500-mL Easy Bag

RTH/Easy Bag/DRIPAC-flex are ready-to-hang presentations. AA, amino acids.

6

Content of parenteral feeds

The aims of this chapter are:

- to describe the usual mode of presentation of parenteral nutrition and explain how it is compounded;
- to describe the main energy and nitrogen sources used in parenteral nutrition;
- to describe the electrolytes, minerals and trace elements used in parenteral nutrition;
- to provide examples of typical regimens used.

Parenteral regimens

The pharmaceutical industry provides a range of pre-compounded admixtures to which vitamins and trace elements are added. Alternatively, the parenteral solutions can be compounded locally in a sterile production unit, or a combination of both methods can be used.

Parenteral regimens are usually administered in 2.5-L bags, and most hospitals have a range of solutions to meet the majority of patient requirements. The bags used to store the PN are now multi-layered and laminated, which is important for minimizing degradation of the light-sensitive vitamins, e.g. vitamin C. Once compounded, these regimens are nutritionally complete.

These all-in-one (AIO) mixtures can contain up to 50 different compounds and are intrinsically unstable. It is therefore essential that the pharmacist ensures not only the stability and compatibility of these complex admixtures, but also their clinical efficacy and safety.

A number of interactions can occur which will compromise the stability of the AIO admixture. They include:

- the physico-chemical stability of the lipid emulsion;
- the chemical stability and incompatibility problems associated with the combination of amino acids and glucose used;
- the precipitation of chemical compounds in the aqueous phase;
- the stability and incompatibility of vitamins, trace elements and any added drugs, e.g. cimetidine, to the AIO admixture.

It is for these reasons that there can be limitations, particularly on electrolyte content, in some PN regimens.

Parenteral solutions are a potential growth medium for bacteria, and hence it is essential that they are compounded under aseptic conditions and that *no additions are made at ward level*. In the UK these aseptic facilities must meet the requirements of good manufacturing practice and the Farwell Report (*Guide to Good Manufacturing Practice for Medical Products*, European Community Commissioner, 1992)

Due to the complexity of the compounding procedures, full details of all parenteral solutions are not listed in this text. The PN pharmacist, who will have the expert knowledge and access to product literature, should be consulted.

Once compounded, the bags can be kept in a designated ward refrigerator at 2–8°C for 6 days, and must be used by day 7 or discarded. If PN bags are left at room temperature for more than 48 h, cracking of the emulsion will occur.

Energy sources

The only energy sources used in parenteral nutrition in the UK are glucose and lipid.

Glucose can be used to provide energy for up to 60 per cent of requirements. The disadvantages of providing glucose in excess of requirements have been discussed in Chapter 2. In addition, septic patients can only utilize 3 mg glucose/kg/min, compared with a healthy individual who can use 5 mg/kg/min (about 2000 kcal/day for a 70-kg man). This is due to the increase in oxygen consumption and myocardial workload in the septic patient. As already mentioned, in the critically ill patient neurohormonal responses will promote hyperglycaemia.

- Administering glucose in excess of the normal hepatic production rate (1–2 mg/kg/min) will exacerbate the problem.
- High circulating glucose levels may impair phagocyte function, which is relevant in septic patients.
- Sustained glucose levels above 12 mmol/L have been shown to impair the chemotactic and phagocytic activity of activated monocytes, and will therefore impede the immune response.

In practice, therefore, a 40 to 60 per cent glucose or 40 to 60 per cent fat mixture is administered.

Fat cannot be administered as a sole energy source (see Chapter 2), and some glucose is needed to utilize fat.

One of the fat sources that can be used in parenteral feeds is Intralipid (10, 20 or 30 per cent), which is a soyabean emulsion, mainly long-chain triglycerides. It also contains 8 per cent omega-3 fatty acids and 59 per cent omega-6 fatty acids. For example, 500 mL of Intralipid (20 per cent) yields 110 g of fat and 999 kcal of energy. This is because 500 mL of Intralipid contain 11 g of glycerol, which provide 99 kcal (1 g of glycerol provides 9 kcal).

There are many other fat sources available on the market, e.g. Lipovenos 10/20 per cent (Fresenius) with a similar composition to Intralipid and Lipofundin MCT/LCT10/20 per cent (Braun), which is 50 per cent soya and 50 per cent MCT.

The advantages of using fat as an energy source in parenteral nutrition are as follows.

- Whole body protein is replenished faster when 15–40 per cent of total energy is provided as fat.
- Although glucose which is not utilized for energy is converted into fat, the yield is 30 per cent less than the theoretical yield from glucose.
- Fat oxidation produces less carbon dioxide.
- The use of fat allows the use of lower osmolality feeds with less vein damage, so they can be used peripherally if required. This reduces the risk of osmotic irritation and phlebitis, allowing some solutions to be administered via a peripheral vein if necessary.
- Fat provides essential fatty acids.

The disadvantages of using fat as an energy source are as follows.

- Abnormal liver function tests – these generally occur after 2–3 weeks on PN, and are usually benign and reversible. However, if the dose exceeds 3 g/kg/day (150–180 g fat/day), steatosis and cholestasis may result and the regimen should be altered accordingly, e.g. use 10 per cent Intralipid rather than 20 per cent (see Chapter 7).

- The cost of fat is 5–7 times that of glucose on a calorie-for-calorie basis.
- Some patients, particularly the critically ill, have problems clearing fat from the plasma (see Chapter 7).

In summary, the dual energy system is more efficient metabolically, so fewer calories are needed for an equal protein-sparing effect.

Energy calculations

The energy provided from fat and glucose sources in PN is usually expressed as non-nitrogen or non-protein energy, the intention being that glucose and fat kilocalories are used for energy and not protein. However, this does not mean that energy from protein oxidation is not used, and it should contribute to final calculations.

Nitrogen sources

The protein source in PN is generally a mixture of essential and non-essential synthetic amino acids. Some amino acid solutions may also contain added glucose, e.g. Nutriflex Basal (Braun) and/or added minerals, e.g. phosphate in FreAmine III 8.5 per cent (Fresenius).

The amount of protein in PN solutions is usually expressed as grams of nitrogen. Therefore, 1 L of Vamin glucose contains 60 g of amino acids, which is equivalent to 9.4 g of nitrogen.

All proteins contain about 16 per cent of nitrogen by weight. Therefore, to convert grams of amino acids to grams of nitrogen:

$$60 \text{ g of amino acids} = \frac{60}{100} \times 16 = 9.6 \text{ g of nitrogen.}$$

To convert grams of nitrogen to grams of protein:

1 g of nitrogen = 6.25 g of protein
Therefore 9.6 g of nitrogen = 60 g of protein.

Currently nitrogen sources in parenteral nutrition consist of free amino acids produced by a variety of companies. These include

Aminoplasmal (Braun), Aminoplex (Geistlich), Clinimix (Nestlé Clinical) and FreAmine (Fresenius).

All companies also provide a range of nitrogen sources to meet varying patient requirements, e.g. Pharmacia provide Vamin glucose (9 g of nitrogen/L), Vamin 14 (13.5 g N_2/L) and Vamin 18 (18 gN_2/L).

There are now some products on the market which are supplemented with the glutamine dipeptide, e.g. Glamin (Pharmacia) and Dipeptiven (Fresenius) supplemented with L-alanyl-L-glutamine, both providing 20 g of glutamine/L.

There are also products supplemented with BCAAs.

Table 6.1 A typical parenteral regimen for a patient with no electrolyte abnormalities or fluid restriction

	Body weight 50 kg	Body weight 70 kg
Nitrogen (g)	9	13.5
Non-protein energy (kcal)	1600	2200
Fluid (L)	2.5	2.5
Sodium (mmol)	80	122.5
Potassium (mmol)	60	80
Calcium (mmol)	5	5
Magnesium (mmol)	7	7
Phosphate (mmol)	28	38

Should fluid/electrolyte/mineral restrictions exist, then there is flexibility to adjust the content to meet requirements.

Electrolyte content of parenteral regimens

Potassium

Parenteral regimens usually provide 60–100 mmol per day of potassium for patients with normal requirements.

Hypokalaemia can be a problem in parenterally fed patients due to the following.

- If amphotericin B, a nephrotoxic drug, is given as part of the antimicrobial regimen in bone marrow transplant patients, there are inevitably large losses of potassium.

- Profuse diarrhoea can cause potassium losses.
- Infusion of large amounts of glucose can precipitate hypokalaemia because, when glucose is transported into the cells under the influence of insulin, potassium is also carried into the cells and is thus removed from the circulation.

Sodium

Regimens usually contain 80–120 mmol per day for patients with normal requirements.

Hypernatraemia can be a common problem in ICU, and can be linked to dehydration.

Mineral content of parenteral regimens

Calcium

Patients on short-term parenteral nutrition probably do not need supplementation, since adequate amounts can be mobilized from the bone.

Normally 5 mmol is included in the feed, which rarely needs to be adjusted.

Magnesium

The main problem is hypomagnesaemia. If levels fall below 0.5 mmol/L the clinical symptoms are cardiac arrhythmias and central nervous system (CNS) effects.

Hypomagnesaemia usually coexists with hypokalaemia and sometimes with hypocalcaemia.

Magnesium (5–10 mmol) is included in feeds, which is sufficient to maintain levels, but if the patient was previously deficient, it is best to administer the magnesium as a separate infusion.

Phosphate

Hypophosphataemia will produce symptoms if the level is < 0.15 mmol/L. They include muscle weakness, bone pain, paraesthesias and impaired functioning of red blood cells (RBCs).

Most regimens provide 20–30 mmol/day.

Vitamins

In practice, one vial of Solivito and one of Vitlipid are included in the compounding of each bag daily. This provides the American Medical Association recommended daily amounts of water-soluble and fat-soluble vitamins, respectively (see Appendix 6.1).

Other vitamin preparations are available, such as Cernevit (Nestlé Clinical), which provides both water- and fat-soluble vitamins in the same preparation, and Multibionta (Baxter), which is not as comprehensive.

Trace elements

These include iron, copper, chromium, manganese, cobalt, selenium, iodine, fluorine, zinc and molybdenum.

Clinical deficiencies of any of these are rare and would normally take several weeks to appear. However, it is not known whether sub-clinical deficiency can occur, particularly in convalescence when requirements may be higher (Okada *et al.*, 1995).

In the short term, zinc deficiency can occur within a period of a few weeks, and can result in impaired wound healing, lethargy and reduced protein synthesis. In certain conditions zinc supplementation is recommended, e.g. patients with large upper gastrointestinal fistulae losses (> 1 L/day) (see Chapter 3).

Both minerals and trace elements can be provided by Addiphos and Additrace, respectively. Both products are manufactured by Pharmacia (see Appendix 6.2).

Case study

A 45-year-old man (weight from ward chart 120 kg, height 1.90 m) is admitted to the ICU with suspected sepsis following collapse at ward level.

- Previous medical history – 2 weeks post-cystectomy and ileal conduit for cancer of the bladder.
- On admission to ICU:
  1. multiple urine leaks, two drains through large and small bowel;
  2. chest infection and respiratory distress;

3. intubated and ventilated.
• Biochemistry shows the following:

urea	14 mmol/L
sodium	140 mmol/L
potassium	4.3 mmol/L
bilirubin	26 μ mol/L
creatinine	194 μ mol/L
calcium	1.92 mmol/L
phosphate	0.77 mmol/L
ALP	161 IU/L
AST	34 IU/L
magnesium	0.92 mmol/L
albumin	24 g/L

• The ICU team have requested 2.5 L of PN for this patient.

1. Calculate this patient's requirements. Consider if you would use actual or ideal body weight for this patient.
2. Calculate a suitable regimen for this patient, containing 2.5 L of fluid as requested, and consider particularly the electrolyte content of the regimen.

In practice, an ideal body weight should be used to calculate this patient's requirements, as he is overweight and the dangers of overfeeding have already been discussed.

In consideration of the regimen most suitable for this patient, the volume and electrolyte content of the regimen chosen will have to be monitored daily from biochemistry and any fluid losses from drains.

References

European Community Commissioners 1992: *Rules governing medicinal products in the European Community. Vol. IV. Guide to good manufacturing practice for medical products.* Commissioners of the European Community.

Okada, A., Takagi, Y., Nezu, R., Sando, K. and Shenkin, A. 1995: Trace element metabolism in parenteral and enteral nutrition. *Nutrition* **11**, 106–13.

Further reading

Pennington, C.R. 1996: Nutritional requirements. In: *Current perspectives on parenteral nutrition in adults*. Biddenden: British Association for Parenteral and Enteral Nutrition, 12–21.

Appendix 6.1

One vial of Solivito provides the recommended daily dose of the following water-soluble vitamins:

Vitamin	Dose	Daily recommended i.v. dose
Vitamin B_1	3.1 mg	3–20 mg
Vitamin B_2	4.9 mg	3–8 mg
Nicotinamide	40 mg	40 mg
Vitamin B_6	4.9 mg	4–6 mg
Pantothenic acid	16.5 mg	10–20 mg
Biotin	60 μg	60 μg
Folic acid	0.4 mg	0.2–0.4 mg
Vitamin B_{12}	5.0 μg	5–15 μg
Vitamin C	100 mg	100 mg

One ampoule of Vitlipid N Adult provides the following daily requirements for fat-soluble vitamins:

Vitamin	Dose	Daily recommended intake
Vitamin A	990 μg	800–2500 μg as retinol or retinol palmitate
Vitamin D	5 μg	5 μg as ergocalciferol
Vitamin E	10 mg	10 mg as alpha-tocopherol

Appendix 6.2

One vial of Addiphos (20 mL) provides the following:

Phosphate	40 mmol
Potassium	30 mmol
Sodium	30 mmol

The volume of Addiphos administered can be varied depending on the patient's individual requirements.

One ampoule of Additrace (10 mL) contains the following trace elements:

Iron	20 μg
Zinc	100 μg
Manganese	5 μg
Copper	20 μg
Chromium	0.2 μg
Selenium	0.4 μg
Molybdenum	0.2 μg
Fluoride	50 μg
Iodide	1 μg

The dosage can be altered if larger amounts are required.

7

How to start feeding

The aims of this chapter are:

- to discuss factors governing the choice of type of nutritional support;
- to outline the steps facilitating problem-free commencement of nutritional support.

Introduction

There is limited evidence to suggest that early commencement of enteral nutrition can influence septic morbidity in particular groups of critically ill patients. Benefits have been shown in abdominal trauma and burns patients (Moore *et al.*, 1989; Kudsk *et al.*, 1992). Other evidence suggests that there are benefits in the form of gastrointestinal protection and possibly support of gastrointestinal immune function (Alverdy *et al.*, 1985; Alverdy, 1990).

Choice of type of nutritional support

This will depend on:

- whether the gut is functioning;
- which route is appropriate;
- how long the patient will be fed for (this is difficult to predict in the majority of ICU patients).

If the gut is functioning, then enteral nutritional support is the preferred method for the reasons listed below:

- preservation of gastrointestinal (GI) tract morphology and function;

- support of the immune function of the GI tract;
- nutritional delivery mirrors normal physiology more closely;
- enteral nutrition is considerably less expensive than parenteral nutrition;
- enteral nutrition is associated with fewer life-threatening complications.

Factors affecting the patient's ability to tolerate enteral nutrition include:

- pre-existing malnutrition;
- elective/emergency surgery;
- medication – opiates, vasopressors;
- Diagnosis.

Enteral nutrition

Nutritional support via the gastrointestinal tract remains the route of choice for critically ill patients. It has clinical, immunological and financial advantages over parenteral nutrition due to its relative ease of administration, lower cost and its association with fewer complications. Enteral nutrition maintains the gut mucosal defence system together with prevention of gut mucosal atrophy (Alverdy *et al.*, 1985, 1988). Septic complications and infectious morbidity are significantly reduced in patients suffering abdominal trauma (Kudsk *et al.*, 1992). While every effort should be made to feed via the enteral route, it is not always possible. The routes for enteral feeding are shown in Fig. 7.1.

Contraindications to enteral nutrition

Absolute contraindications include:

- complete gastrointestinal dysfunction due to multiple organ failure;
- prolonged paralytic ileus;
- gastrointestinal fistulae situated in or distal to the jejunum;
- short gut syndrome (< 100 cm of residual jejunum).

Relative contraindications include:

- upper gastrointestinal obstruction;

- malabsorption syndromes;
- pancreatitis.

An enteral nutrition algorithm is shown in Fig. 7.2.

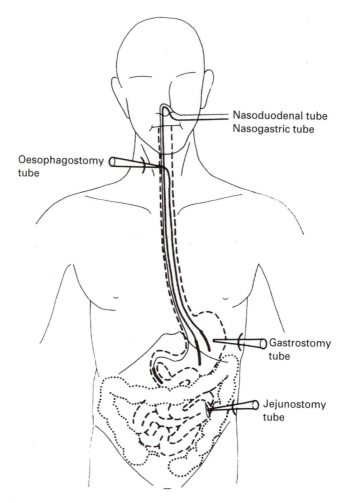

Fig. 7.1 Diagrammatic representation of routes for enteral feeding. Reproduced with kind permission of Blackwell Science from Thomas: *Manual of dietetic practice*. 2nd edn. p. 67. Blackwell Science.

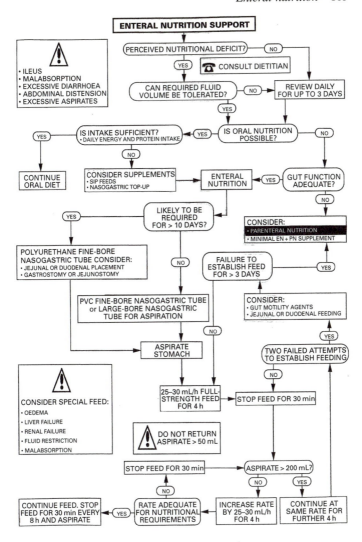

Fig. 7.2 Enteral nutrition algorithm. Adapted from Armstrong, R.F., Bullen, C., Cohen S.L., Singer, M. and Webb, A. 1991: *Critical care algorithms*. Oxford: Oxford University Press.

Starter regimen

Enteral feeding can begin as soon as the patient is admitted to the intensive care unit. Full-strength feeds should always be used when commencing a patient on enteral feed, as there is no evidence that the use of water and half-strength feed makes any difference to tolerance (Adam and Batson, 1997). The use of full-strength feed allows progression to appropriate levels of protein and energy intake as early as possible. In addition, attempts to add water to sterile feeds increase the risk of bacterial contamination and diarrhoea (Keohane *et al.*, 1984; Anderton, 1993).

It may be necessary to administer feed at a slow rate initially and to increase to full-volume requirements over a 12- to 48-h period depending on the patient's ability to tolerate feed. This will be of particular importance if the patient has not had any oral intake for more than 2–3 days.

Administration rate

There is no doubt that administering full-strength feeds at too fast a rate can be detrimental to the patient. The administration rate will depend on the volume prescribed to meet nutritional requirements, the unit policy regarding rest periods to allow gastric pH to normalize, the patient's tolerance (physical or psychological), his or her medical condition, and how frequently interruptions for investigations or procedures occur. The speed with which the rate of feeding is increased will depend on the patient's tolerance and sometimes on local policy.

Aspiration and measurement of gastric residual contents are commonly used as an indicator of tolerance. There is little published work to establish the point at which high volumes of gastric aspirate become significant. However, McClave *et al.* (1992) found, in a study comparing healthy individuals with critically ill patients, that 200-mL cut-off volumes would effectively identify gastric intolerance whilst ensuring that the healthy gut would continue to be fed. These researchers also pointed out that single high volumes of gastric aspirate were rarely significant markers of intolerance. If gastric aspirates are greater than 200 mL on three consecutive occasions at 4-hourly intervals, then alternative measures such as gastric motility stimulants or naso/jejunal/duodenal feeding should be considered.

If the introduction of enteral nutrition is unsuccessful and parenteral nutrition is required, enteral nutrition should not be abandoned completely. Unless absolutely contraindicated, a minimal amount of feed (e.g. 25–30 mL/h) should be administered in order to supply the gut.

In the early stages of this fine tuning, the absence of bowel sounds is not an absolute indicator of gastric intolerance, and attempts to feed should continue unless they are accompanied by other signs of gastrointestinal dysfunction. These include vomiting, abdominal pain and/or distension, and uncontrollable diarrhoea.

Overnight enteral feeding

Where patients are only managing a minimal oral intake and further nutrients are required, it is useful to consider feeding overnight in order to supplement daily intake. Appetite is not affected during the day when oral intake can be encouraged; however, nutritional goals can still be met.

Stopping an enteral feed

Ideally, there should be a transitional period between enteral nutrition and return to an oral diet. During this time the quantity of feed is gradually reduced as oral intake improves. This ensures that nutritional intake is not compromised. During this transition, accurate records of oral intake are invaluable in helping the dietitian to assess when a patient no longer requires enteral nutrition. In practice, feeding can usually be stopped once the patient has reached the goal of 1000 kcal/day or 50 per cent of his or her nutritional requirement.

Types of enteral feeding tubes

Nasogastric tubes

This is the most common route, and provides immediate access to the stomach in an acute situation.

Ryle's tubes: These are primarily used for aspiration of the stomach and no longer have a place in long-term tube feeding. The tubes are made from PVC, and complications associated with their use are now well documented. In addition it has been reported that they render the lower oesophageal sphincter incompetent, thus increasing the risk of gastric reflux (Cataldi-Betcher *et al.*, 1983;

Taylor, 1988; Williams, 1992). This has recently been disputed by Dotson *et al.* (1994), who showed that the size of the nasogastric tube is not an important determinant of gastric reflux during short-term intubation of normal subjects. This does not necessarily extend to critically ill patients receiving mechanical ventilation. It has also been suggested that large-bore tubes tend to interfere with coughing and spontaneous respiration (Cataldi-Betcher *et al.*, 1983);

Complications associated with the use of Ryle's tubes include:

- mucosal irritation;
- oesophageal ulceration;
- oesophageal perforation;
- sinusitis;
- tracheo-oesophageal fistula.

Fine-bore feeding tubes: These are nasogastric tubes with an internal lumen of 1–2 mm or French gauge 6–9 (1 FR (French) = 0.33 mm). They are made from PVC, polyurethane or silicone. They are softer, more pliable and generally more comfortable for the patient than a Ryle's tube, and are less likely to cause complications, although these may still occur. Complications, which are often due to poor knowledge and insertion technique, include:

- tracheal and pleural intubation;
- tube misplacement;
- oesophageal perforation (Metheny *et al.*, 1988b).

PVC fine-bore tubes have a maximum life of 10 days, and are only occasionally used in the critically ill patient. The slightly more rigid properties of PVC mean that a guidewire is not necessary for insertion, e.g. Flexiflow (Cow and Gate) 8 FR PVC tube without guidewire for short-term use.

Polyurethane or silicone tubes have a maximum lifespan of 3–6 months. They are used more frequently in the critically ill patient, thus avoiding the repetitive trauma associated with the frequent changes necessary with a PVC tube. They are recommended for the intensive care setting, e.g. Flexiflow (Cow and Gate) 8 FR polyurethane tube with guidewire for long-term use, or Silk (Merck) 6/8 FR silicone tube with guidewire for long-term use.

The internal diameter of the silicone tube is actually smaller than that of the polyurethane tube, and this has been associated with an increased incidence of clogging (Metheny *et al.*, 1988a).

A recently developed nasogastric tube specially designed to re-duce the frequency of obstruction (Radius International) has been shown to have a greatly reduced incidence of obstruction, as well as being significantly easier to place (Silk *et al.*, 1996).

Smaller size tubes are the choice in critically ill patients, as minimal nasal obstruction and a reduced incidence of ulceration are desirable.

Contrary to some reports, it is possible and often necessary to feed a patient nasogastrically if he or she is receiving long-term oxygen via a face mask or nasal cannulae.

Enteral nutrition should always be considered when CPAP is required. It is beneficial in those patients who are unable to maintain their nutritional intake due to fatigue or dependence on the CPAP. It will reduce the discomfort and potential danger (increased risk of pulmonary aspiration) associated with air swallowing as a result of the high gas flows and the positive pressure.

Nasojejunal and nasoduodenal tubes

These are fine-bore feeding tubes which are longer than 110 cm and made of polyurethane. Some are also weighted to aid transpyloric passage into the small bowel. They may be the tube of choice when commencing feeding in a patient who is at high risk of oesophageal reflux or in whom gastric stasis is likely. However, transpyloric passage can be difficult to achieve and endoscopy is the preferred method of insertion (Lewis *et al.*, 1990; Baskin and Johanson, 1995), e.g. Medicina (7 FR) polyurethane tube with guidewire and weight for long-term use, Corsafe (8 FR) polyurethane tube with guidewire and weight for long-term use, or Silk (8 FR) polyurethane tube with guidewire, unweighted for long-term use.

Both Corsafe and Medicina tubes require placement by endoscopy. Recently, a self-propelling nasoenteric feeding tube has been introduced with apparent success (Jeppson *et al.*, 1992). It consists of a fine-bore silicone tube with five loops at the distal end. The loops are straightened out by a guidewire during insertion, but reshape following removal of the guidewire. Peristalsis moves the loops forward, promoting pyloric passage and movement into the jejunum, e.g. Flocare Bengmark (8 and 10 FR) Nutricia silicone tube with guidewire for long-term use.

Gastrostomy

Percutaneous endoscopic gastrostomy (PEG): This consists of a transabdominal feeding tube which is inserted by endoscopy under local anaesthetic and intravenous sedation. The procedure can be undertaken either in the endoscopy unit or in the ICU itself. Experienced medical personnel are required to carry out the procedure with the assistance of nurses trained in endoscopy and/or nutrition nurse specialists.

Percutaneous endoscopic gastrostomy is now the technique of choice for long-term feeding (Peters and Westaby, 1994), and should be considered if feeding is required for longer than a 4-week period. It is often more comfortable and cosmetically more acceptable for the aware patient than a nasogastric tube. The PEG tube is made from either polyurethane or silicone, e.g. the Freka PEG system – Charriere (CH) 9 and 15 (Fresenius) – has a maximum life span of 18 months, and the Bower PEG system – CH 12 and 20 (Merck) – has a maximum life span of 1–2 years.

Contraindications for PEG include:

- oesophageal varices;
- peritonitis;
- peritoneal dialysis;
- massive ascites;
- severe gastro-oesophageal reflux;
- previous recent gastrointestinal surgery, e.g. oesophagostomy or oesophagogastrectomy;
- gastric outlet obstruction;
- significant uncorrectable coagulation disorders.

In general, the vast majority of critically ill patients requiring enteral nutrition continue to be fed via nasogastric tubes (98 per cent; Adam and Batson, 1997), although the incidence of PEG usage has increased.

Surgically placed gastrostomy: is the traditional method of placement, which requires a general anaesthetic and a laparotomy. A 'fistula' tract between the stomach and the abdominal surface is created. This type of tube insertion is rarely used in the critically ill patient unless preceded by major gastrointestinal surgery. Examples include silicone surgical gastrostomy tube CH 12–24 (Sherwood), which has a maximum life span of 1–3 months, and the silicone urinary catheter, with a maximum life span 4–6 weeks.

In **gastrostomy placed under ultrasound guidance**, a transabdominal feeding tube is placed under ultrasound guidance by a radiologist using only local anaesthesia, e.g. percutaneous gastrostomy (maximum life span 6 months to 1 year).

Jejunostomy

Percutaneous endoscopic jejunostomy: A transabdominal feeding tube is inserted by endoscopy under local anaesthetic and i.v. sedation. As with PEGs, this is the technique of choice if feeding is likely to continue for longer than 4 weeks. It is preferable for patients who are at risk of aspiration due to gastric stasis or oesophageal reflux. The tubes themselves are made of polyurethane or silicone, but are longer than the standard gastrostomy tube in order to bypass the stomach and enter the small bowel. This is achieved by piercing the stomach wall with an introducer, passing the tube into the stomach and feeding the tube into the duodenum or jejunum with the aid of an endoscope. *Note* The jejunum is not pierced directly.

Examples include the Freka PEG system CH 9 and 15 intestinal tube (Fresenius) (maximum life span of 6 months to 1 year) and the Bower PEG system with Silk jejunostomy tube CH 20 (Merck) (maximum life span of 1–2 years).

Gastrojejunostomy placed under ultrasound guidance: These are transabdominal feeding tubes inserted using ultrasound guidance under local anaesthetic. This procedure is usually carried out by a radiologist.

Methods of enteral delivery

Delivery of feed can be continuous, intermittent or bolus.

Continuous feeding

Feed is delivered continuously over the 24-h period, with breaks only for aspiration checks or procedures.

Intermittent feeding

Feed is delivered over a period of 18–20 h, with a rest period of between 4–6 h each day. It is thought to reduce the incidence of nosocomial pneumonia (see pages 112–113).

Bolus feeding

Feed is delivered as a small number of high-volume boluses given at times roughly equating to meals. This method most closely reflects 'normal' food intake.

Three main methods are used in the different contexts.

Pump-assisted delivery

A mains-operated or battery-run feeding pump is used to deliver feed either continuously or intermittently. The method of choice for the critically ill patient is continuous pump-assisted delivery. It allows for versatility, flexibility and accuracy of flow rate (see page 113).

Gravity-assisted delivery

A reservoir of feed is hung above the patient and delivered via a giving set with a roller clamp to allow regulation of the rate of delivery. This can be either continuous or intermittent.

Bolus feeding via a syringe

A large volume of feed (usually 25–30 per cent of daily requirements) is administered manually using a syringe.

Advantages and disadvantages of the continuous method of feeding (gravity or pump-assisted)

Continuous feeding is associated with a lower risk of gastrointestinal complications (Williams, 1992). It is less likely to be associated with gastro-oesophageal reflux and malabsorption than bolus delivery of large volumes of feed periodically. However, Dive *et al.* (1994) and Raimundo *et al.* (1989) have shown that continuous delivery of feed intragastrically in critically ill and hospital patients does not interrupt fasting patterns of motility. These patterns include migrating motor complexes which are highly propulsive in nature and may force food through the small intestine at too fast a rate for optimal absorption. This could reduce the ability of the patient to absorb feed and/or reabsorb water, and increase the likelihood of diarrhoea. However, the causal evidence remains scanty, and further research is required.

Continuous feeding into the duodenum does not show this effect (Raimundo *et al.*, 1989), and this is the optimal method of delivering feed into the small intestine. It has also been suggested (Jacobs, 1990; Lee *et al.*, 1990) that continuous enteral delivery is associated with an increased risk of pneumonia due to the alkalinization of the gastric environment, allowing overgrowth of micro-organisms. They found that a period without feeding each day allowed the gastric pH to return to normal, which discouraged bacterial overgrowth. Their findings have yet to be replicated in a large randomized, controlled trial, although intermittent delivery is used in many centres. Bolus methods of feeding are also more likely to be associated with gastrointestinal complications, particularly where large volumes are delivered to patients with reduced gastric motility, and they are rarely used in the critically ill patient.

Pump-assisted feeding

There are two types of pumps, differentiated by their pumping mechanism:

- rotary peristaltic pump;
- bellows cassette.

Rotary peristaltic pump

This type of pump is relatively inexpensive to purchase and easy to control. The administration sets are either one-piece PVC tubing or a silicone tube pumping insert in a PVC set. The advantage of this type of pump is that the same administration set can be used for gravity feeding when required. This option may be useful if pumps are not available. Examples include the Sherwood medical K234 pump and the Ross Laboratories Flexiflow Patrol pump.

Bellows cassette pump

This mechanism is possibly more accurate than the peristaltic pump. It delivers far more consistent volumes and, when fully compressed, gives the prescribed amount to be delivered. The flow rate is determined by the number of compressions per unit time. It cannot be used for gravity feeding. Examples include the Ross Laboratories Companion pump.

Automatic flush pumps

An optional hourly flush system is a recent addition to the range of enteral feed pumps available. If tube obstruction is a problem or additional hydration is required, the pump can be set up to deliver both flush and feed during each hour. Examples include the Ross Laboratories Flexiflow Quantum pump.

Performance criteria for an enteral feed pump for the critically ill

Auty (1994) has defined the criteria for adequate pump performance in the critically ill as follows:

- mains powered with rechargeable battery back-up;
- digital selection of delivery rate in increments of 1 mL/h over a range of 1–300 mL/h;
- preselection of dose volume to a maximum of 3000 mL;
- display of (1) delivery rate, (2) preset dose volume and (3) volume delivered;
- audible and visual alarms for occlusion, end of feed, equipment failure and low battery levels;
- accuracy to within ±10 per cent measured over 1-h periods with consistent output;
- pump inserts to be non-reversible, preventing incorrect loading;
- pumping mechanism capable of pumping water as well as feed for hydration;
- electrical and mechanical design to comply with BS5724 Part 1 (1989) or 1EC601-1;
- electronic design to include watchdog or similar circuitry to monitor integrity of systems and sensors;
- pump to be pole mounted (patient mobility not a consideration).

Administration sets

Sets with roller clamps and flow-rate controllers are widely available from numerous nutrition companies. All types of administration set perform the same basic function, are supplied in sterile packaging, and vary only in cost and design. However, two particular types are associated with a reduction in the incidence of feed contamination.

Integral bag and giving set

The integral bag and giving set system is the preferred alternative to a separate bottle/reservoir system, thereby reducing the incidence of bacterial contamination which is often associated with enteral feed systems (Anderton, 1993).

Ready-to-hang systems

The 'ready-to-hang' concept (i.e. with the feed in a container which is used as the reservoir for feeding) has reduced the incidence of contamination still further by minimizing handling and the opportunity for direct contact with the feed.

It is important to remember the following key points when starting to feed.

- When the gut is functioning, always feed enterally.
- Consider the need for feed within 6–12 h of admission.
- Use a standard feed from the start – pre-diluted feeds are unnecessary.
- Use the appropriate material/size of feeding tube.
- Check gastric emptying prior to commencing the feed.
- Commence feeding at a low rate and aspirate after 4 h.
- Increase the rate of feeding as tolerated.
- Aim to achieve the feed volume/calorie goal within a 24-h period.

Parenteral nutrition

A parenteral nutrition (PN) algorithm is shown in Fig. 7.3. Traditional high-osmolarity parenteral nutrition is administered through a central venous catheter into either the internal or external jugular vein, the subclavian or the cephalic veins. The catheter tip should sit at the junction of the superior vena cava and the right atrium. PN is administered via these routes due to the high osmolarity and viscous nature of the feed, which would cause severe trauma to smaller, peripheral veins. Unfortunately the administration of central vein parenteral nutrition is not without its problems (potential complications such as central vein thrombosis, pneumothorax and infection are outlined and explained in Chapter 8).

In the intensive-care unit, parenteral nutrition will be administered either through a dedicated lumen of a triple-lumen catheter or via a

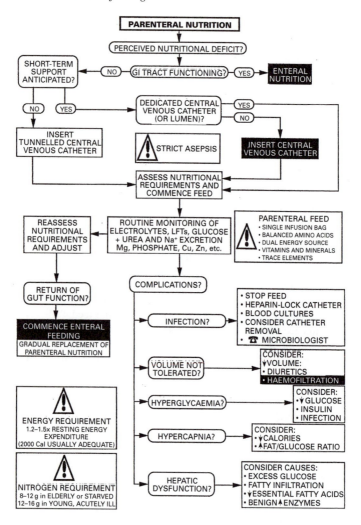

Fig. 7.3 Parenteral nutrition algorithm (reproduced with permission from Armstrong, R.F., Bullen, C., Cohen, S.L., Singer, M. and Webb, A. 1991: *Critical care alogrithms.* Oxford: Oxford University Press).

single-lumen (usually tunnelled) central venous catheter. The tunnelled catheter is a technique which utilizes the skin of the patient as a bacterial defence against catheter contamination, and is less frequently associated with catheter-related infection in the long-term patient.

Tunnelled catheters

Due to the high risk of infection associated with parenteral nutrition solutions, it is important that these types of central venous catheters are inserted in a strict sterile environment, e.g. theatre. However, it is common practice in the ICU for tunnelled catheters to be inserted at the bedside. Ideally, insertion should be carried out where there are imaging facilities available, and by highly experienced clinicians or specially trained nutrition nurse specialists.

The tunnelled technique was initially used in an attempt to reduce the incidence of catheter infection, but this can only be achieved if insertion and manipulation of the catheter are undertaken by specially trained personnel following strict hospital policy. However, it is debatable whether the incidence of infection in tunnelled lines is significantly different to that of multi-lumen catheters, although the life span of a tunnelled catheter has been reported to be longer than that of other types of catheter (Keohane *et al.*, 1983; Moran *et al.*, 1987; Payne James *et al.*, 1989).

Tunnelling of catheters does make it easier and more convenient for the catheter to be manipulated, the site dressed and the catheter secured, all of which contribute significantly to a decreased likelihood of infection or dislodgement over a long period of time.

Types of tunnelled catheter

Choice is made according to the expected duration of feeding. In cases where patients are aware, they may express their own views regarding comfort and acceptability.

1. A central venous catheter without a cuff is primarily used for medium- to long-term duration, i.e. an anticipated maximum of 3 months. This type of catheter is secured by sutures at the exit site and can be removed easily. Examples include the Nutricath 11 SWG/18 SWG (standard wire gauge) non-cuffed silicone line and the Viggo secalon 16g non-cuffed polyurethane line.
2. A central venous catheter with a Dacron cuff is used in long-term feeding, i.e. when the anticipated duration of feeding is longer than 3 months. This type of catheter is held in place in its subcutaneous tunnel by a Dacron cuff/fibrous sheath that self-

adheres to the tunnel and thereby reduces dislodgement and migration of bacteria from exit to entry site. Removal of the catheter is by careful dissection. Examples include the Hickman 12 FR/9 FR cuffed silicone line and the cuff Cath 14g/16g cuffed polyurethane line. The life span of these catheters is up to and beyond 6 months.

Non-tunnelled catheters

Multi-lumen central venous catheters are not tunnelled catheters. They are inserted in a similar manner to tunnelled lines, with the catheter tip sitting at the junction of the superior vena cava and right atrium. Their position is confirmed by chest X-ray (CXR). Multi-lumen catheters are of benefit to patient, clinician and nurse in the intensive-care setting. They will have up to four lumens, which is increasingly necessary for the administration of intravenous fluids, drugs, blood and colloid, parenteral nutrition and other infusions, as well as for central venous pressure monitoring.

These catheters are potentially susceptible to the same complications as single-lumen catheters. It is common practice to dedicate one lumen for PN only. All other lumens on the catheter should be cared for as meticulously as the PN lumen in order to avoid infection and trauma. Recently, some catheters have been impregnated with chlorhexidine and silver sulphadiazine to reduce further the risk of infection (Pennington, 1996).

A wealth of documentation has been published on the debate surrounding the use of these types of lines for PN, particularly in relation to the incidence of catheter-related infection (McCarthy *et al.*, 1987; Clarke-Christoff *et al.*, 1992).

Research studies aimed at ending this uncertainty have resulted in the publication of many conflicting reports. Clarke-Christoff *et al.* (1992) reported that 78 patients randomized to either a single-lumen or a triple-lumen catheter showed a significantly lower incidence of catheter-related sepsis in the single-lumen group. Rodrigo *et al.* (1989) reported no significant difference in the incidence of catheter-related sepsis between single- and triple-lumen catheter groups in a trial of 145 critically ill patients.

The decision regarding catheter type should be based on clinical experience, research where possible, and local hospital policies and protocols.

Peripheral parenteral nutrition (PPN)

The critically ill patient will usually receive PN via a central line because access is invariably already present, and there are often fluid-volume limitations. In addition, the level of nutritional requirement frequently cannot be met by peripheral parenteral nutrition solutions. However, in a few patients this method may have potential benefits. Centrally delivered PN is being used less and less in general ward patients, and there is now evidence that PPN is undoubtedly the route of choice in this group (Madan *et al.*, 1992; Everitt *et al.*, 1993). This is because the advantages of PPN benefit both the patient and the clinician. There are certain circumstances within the intensive-care unit where PPN could be successfully used (Payne James, 1993). The patient must require less than 14 g of nitrogen and less than 2000 kcal of energy per day. They should have no limitation on fluid intake, and be able to tolerate relatively high levels of lipid (more than 50 per cent of non-protein calories) (Powell-Tuck, 1978).

The benefits of peripheral intravenous nutrition delivery include:

- relative ease of access;
- simple insertion technique;
- reduced costs;
- reduced incidence of complications.

The limitations of PPN in general patients were seen as hyper-osmolarity, high fluid volumes limiting delivery of patient requirements, and a frequent incidence of thrombophlebitis. The volume and osmolarity of PPN solutions have changed considerably over the last few years. The widespread use of lipid emulsions together with carbohydrate as an energy source has reduced the osmolarity of the feeds, and new developments in cannula design and materials have played a significant part in reducing the incidence of thrombo-phlebitis (Colagiovanni *et al.*, 1996). Bearing these factors in mind, the administration of PPN in the critically ill patient may now be a viable proposition for some intensive-care patients.

Precise knowledge of the catheter insertion technique, appropriate feeding catheters and subsequent nursing care is essential. Catheter longevity can be increased and the incidence of thrombophlebitis reduced if the following adjuncts are used: heparin, hydrocortisone and GTN (see Chapter 8). It is therefore possible to maintain a single catheter throughout the whole course of PPN. This undoubtedly avoids many of the complications associated with central venous parenteral nutrition.

Patient selection – exclusion criteria

PPN should not be used in patients who have:

1. calorie or protein requirements that are greater than can be safely supplied by PPN, e.g.:

   - fluid restriction of < 2000 mL/day;
   - high energy requirements of > 2000 kcal/day;
   - nitrogen requirements of > 14 g/day;

2. lipid intolerance;
3. high or unusual electrolyte requirements;
4. no suitable peripheral veins, i.e. they are inadequate or inaccessible.

Patient selection – inclusion criteria

1. The relevant central veins are thrombosed, or prospective insertion sites are infected by injury or surgery.
2. There is an increased risk of fungal or bacterial sepsis, e.g. in patients with purulent tracheostomy secretions, immune deficiency states or a history of repeated septic episodes.

Methods of administration of PPN

There are three methods of administering PPN:

- administration through a ported cannula;
- cyclical rotation of the cannula site;
- administration through a fine-bore neonatal catheter.

Administration through a ported catheter

Venous access can be obtained using a small and short Teflon-coated intravenous cannula. Unfortunately, the material for the main part of the cannula is PVC – a rigid material which significantly increases the incidence of peripheral vein thrombophlebitis (PVT). It is therefore not surprising that these cannulae require removal and resiting after 24–48 h when PVT is evident or suspected (Madan *et al.*, 1992). They are commonly sited in the hand or proximal forearm.

The choice of access site, coupled with the use of rigid material, proves unpopular and uncomfortable for the patient.

Cyclical rotation of the cannula site

Some experts advocate the use of the above, but choose electively to remove it after each infusion (Pennington, 1996). It is therefore preferable that cannulation sites are identified in both arms. The use of this method has also been shown to be an important factor in reducing thrombophlebitis, although in practical terms it is labour intensive, and repeated cannulations are distressing for the patient (Kevin *et al.*, 1991). It is dependent on the availability of a nutrition nurse specialist or intravenous specialist at the appropriate time of day. This method therefore cannot be recommended.

The cannula type is a Teflon intravenous catheter, 18–20 g in diameter and 2–3.5 cm in length, e.g. Venflon (Ohmeda). This is for short-term use, i.e. 1–4 days.

Administration through a fine-bore neonatal catheter (22–23 gauge)

This is now the technique of choice for the administration of PPN. It was first described by Kolhardt (Kolhardt *et al.*, 1991). Since then, much research has been undertaken to establish its efficacy (Khawajia *et al.*, 1991; Madan *et al.*, 1992). There is now a general consensus that the use of a neonatal-sized venous catheter in a peripheral vein of an adult significantly reduces the incidence of thrombophlebitis compared to the use of short-stay peripheral intravenous catheters (Madan *et al.*, 1992; Everitt *et al.*, 1993).

The type of material and the small gauge directly influence the results. They are responsible for:

- less trauma to the epithelial lining of the peripheral vein;
- a lower capacity for platelet adherence – with reduced risk of thrombosis formation;
- reduced contact.

Increasingly, many centres now use this type of catheter, inserting it into either the basilic or cephalic veins of the arm, or the antecubital fossa. Although initially more expensive than other peripheral cannulae, they are ultimately cheaper in terms of longevity, comfort for the patient and decreased staff time.

The cannula type is a fine-bore polyurethane catheter, 22–23 g in diameter and 15–20 cm in length, e.g. Hydrocath (Ohmeda) and Epicutaneo-cava catheter (Vygon). These are for long-term use up to and beyond 14 days.

Administration equipment

Pump-assisted delivery

PN is only ever administered by one method – pump assisted. Gravity feeding could lead to the administration of a large bolus of PN which could potentially be fatal. In view of this possibility, PN should be administered by a volumetric infusion pump which allows for an accurate delivery of nutrients. Volumetric pumps are fitted with 'occlusion' and 'air-in-line' alarms which do not allow free flow and which use relatively low-cost administration sets, e.g. IVAC 560 series, model 572 or 597, and IMED Gemini PC-1, PC-2 or PC-4.

Administration sets

These are made from silicone, and must have luer-lock connections incorporated into their design. They should be changed with each new bag of PN and should be used for no longer than 24 h. Connections (i.e. extension lines used additionally with the administration set) should be kept to a minimum and also changed regularly, according to local hospital policy, in order to prevent infection and reduce repeated clamping, as this may damage the extension tubing.

Closed luer-lock connection devices

Many centres now use closed luer-lock connection devices, which consist of a protective hub/barrel and silicone membrane. This allows access to the catheter whilst maintaining a closed system and thereby reducing the risk of infection. However, this is not a substitute for quality nursing care in terms of line management and catheter care.

Closed luer-lock systems together with extension lines should be changed weekly, whenever they are damaged, or if blood flashback has occurred. Examples include Bionector – Vygon.

All-in-one bags

PN continues to be supplied in 2.5-L bags which can be administered over a 12- to 48-h period. Within this time limit many patients benefit, in terms of psychological and physiological well-being, from cyclical infusions. However, continuous infusion rates are more appropriate for critically ill patients, particularly those with an irregular fluid load, unstable blood sugar levels or highly variable metabolic responses.

Any additions that need to be made to the bag once it has been sealed should not be made at ward level but in pharmacy, thereby reducing the risk of contamination and incompatibility. Compounded bags of PN should always be stored in a designated refrigerator and removed approximately 2 h before use. If PN does not have sufficient lipid within the bag to provide opacity to ultraviolet light, then it must be protected from the sunlight by covering the bag and thereby preventing the degradation of vitamin A (see Chapter 9).

References

Adam, S. and Batson, S. 1997: A study of problems associated with the delivery of enteral feed in critically ill patients in five ICUs in the UK. *Intensive Care Medicine* **23**, 261–6.

Alverdy, J., Chi, H.S. and Sheldon, G.F. 1985: The effect of parenteral nutrition on gastrointestinal immunity. *Annals of Surgery* **202**, 681–4.

Alverdy, J.C. 1990: Effects of glutamine-supplemented diets on immunology of the gut. *Journal of Parenteral and Enteral Nutrition* **14**, 109S–113S.

Alverdy, J.C., Aoys, E. and Moss, G.S. 1988: Total parenteral nutrition promotes bacterial translocation from the gut. *Surgery* **104**, 185–90.

Anderton, A.L. 1993: Bacterial contamination of enteral feeds and feeding systems. *Clinical Nutrition* **12**, S16–S32.

Auty, B. 1994: Pumps for enteral feeding of critically ill patients. In Rennie, M. (ed.), *Intensive care Britain*, 4th edn. London: Greycoat Publishing, 78–9.

Baskin, W.N. and Johanson, J.F. 1995: An improved approach to delivery of enteral nutrition in the intensive care unit. *Gastrointestinal Endoscopy* **42**, 161–5.

Cataldi-Betcher, E.L., Seltzer, M.H., Slocum, B.A. and Jones, K.W. 1983: Complications occurring during enteral nutrition support. A prospective study. *Journal of Parenteral and Enteral Nutrition* **7**, 546–52.

Colagiovanni, L. 1996: Peripheral benefits. *Nursing Times* **92**, 59–64.

Clarke-Christoff, N., Watters, V.A., Sparks, W., Snyder, B.A. and Grant, J.P. 1992. Use of triple-lumen subclavian catheters for administration of total parenteral nutrition. *Journal of Parenteral and Enteral Nutrition* **16**, 403–7.

Dive, A., Miesse, C., Jamart, J., Evrard, P., Gonzalez, M. and Installe, E.T. 1994: Duodenal motor response to continuous enteral feeding is impaired in mechanically ventilated critically ill patients. *Clinical Nutrition* **13**, 302–6.

Dotson, R.G., Robinson, R.G. and Pingleton, S.K. 1994: Gastro-esophageal reflux with nasogastric tubes: effect of tube sizes. *American Journal of Respiratory and Critical Care Medicine* **149**, 1659–62.

Everitt, N., Madan, M., Alexander, D. and McMahon, M. 1993: Fine bore silicone rubber and polyurethane catheters for the delivery of complete intravenous nutrition via a peripheral vein. *Clinical Nutrition* **12**, 261–5.

Heyland, D.K., Cook, D., Winder, B. and Guyatt, G. 1996: Do critically ill patients tolerate early intragastric enteral nutrition? *Clinical Intensive Care* **7**, 68–73.

Jacobs, S. 1990: Continuous enteral feeding: a major cause of pneumonia among ventilated intensive care patients. *Journal of Parenteral and Enteral Nutrition* **14**, 353–6.

Jeppson, B., Tranberg, K.-G. and Bengmark, S. 1992: Technical developments. A new self-propelling nasoenteric feeding tube. *Clinical Nutrition* **11**, 373–5.

Keohane, P., Attrill, H., Northover, J. *et al.* 1983: Effect of tunnelling and nutrition nurse on catheter sepsis during parenteral nutrition. *Lancet* **12**, 1388–90.

Keohane, P.P., Attrill, H., Love, M., Frost, P. and Silk, D.B.A. 1984: Relation between osmolality of diet and gastrointestinal side-effects in enteral nutrition. *British Medical Journal* **288**, 678–80.

Kevin, M., Pickford, I., Jaegar, H., Couse, N., Mitchell, C. and Maefie, J. 1991: A prospective and randomised study comparing the incidence of infusion phlebitis during continuous and cyclic peripheral parenteral nutrition. *Clinical Nutrition* **10**, 315–9.

Khawajia, H., Williams, J. and Weaver, P. 1991: Transdermal glyceryltrinitrate to allow peripheral total parenteral nutrition: a double-blind placebo-controlled feasibility study. *Journal of the Royal Society of Medicine* **84**, 69–72.

Kolhardt, S.R., Smith, R.C. and Wright, C.R. 1991: Peripheral versus central intravenous nutrition: a comparison of two delivery systems. *British Journal of Surgery* **81**, 67–70.

Kudsk, K.A., Groce, M.A., Fabian, T.C. *et al.* 1992: Enteral versus parenteral feeding: effects on septic morbidity after blunt and penetrating abdominal trauma. *Annals of Surgery* **215**, 503–11.

Lee, B., Chang, R.W.S. and Jacobs, S. 1990: Intermittent nasogastric feeding: a simple and effective method to reduce pneumonia among ventilated ICU patients. *Clinical Intensive Care* **1**, 100–2.

Lewis, B., Maver, K. and Bush, A. 1990: The rapid replacement of jejunal feeding tubes, the Seldinger technique applied to the gut. *Gastrointestinal Endoscopy* **36**, 139–41.

McCarthy, M.C., Shives, J.K., Robison, R.J. and Broadie, T.A. 1987: Prospective evaluation of single and triple lumen catheters on total parenteral nutrition. *Journal of Parenteral and Enteral Nutrition* **11**, 259–62.

McClave, S., Snider, H.L., Lowen, D.D. *et al.* 1992: Use of residual volume as a marker for enteral feeding intolerance: prospective blinded comparison with physical examination and radiographic findings. *Journal of Parenteral and Enteral Nutrition* **16**, 99–105.

Madan, M.I., Alexander D.J. and McMahon, M. 1992: Influence of catheter type on occurrence of thrombophlebitis during peripheral intravenous nutrition. *Lancet* **339**, 101–3.

Metheny, N.A., Eisenberg, P. and McSweeney, M. 1988a: Effect of feeding tube properties and three irrigants on clogging rates. *Nursing Research* **37**, 165–9.

Metheny, N.A., Spies, M.A. and Eisenberg, P. 1988b: Measures to test placement of nasoenteral feeding tubes. *Western Journal of Nursing Research* **10**, 367–83.

Moore, F.A., Moore, E.E. and Jones, T.N. 1989: TEN vs. TPN following abdominal trauma: reduced septic morbidity. *Journal of Trauma* **29**, 916–23.

Moore, F.A., Moore, E.E. and Haenel, J.B. 1995: Clinical benefits of early postinjury feeding. *Clinical Intensive Care* **6**, 21–7.

Moran, K., McEnkee, G., Jones, B., Hone, R., Duigan, J. and O'Malley, E. 1987: To tunnel or not to tunnel catheters for parenteral nutrition. *Annals of the Royal College of Surgeons of England* **69**, 235–6.

Payne-James, J.J. 1993: Peripheral parenteral nutrition: what peripheral vein thrombophlebitis (PVT) prophylaxis to use? In *Intensive Care Britain*. London: Greycoat Publishing, 15–22.

Payne-James, J.J., Grimble, G.K., Rees, R.G. and Silk, D.B.A. 1989: Total parenteral nutrition: clinical applications. *Intensive Therapy and Clinical Monitoring* **January**, 19–26.

Pennington, C.R. 1996: *Current perspectives on parenteral nutrition in adults*. Biddenden: British Association of Parenteral and Enteral Nutrition.

Peters, R.A. and Westaby, D. 1994: Percutaneous endoscopic gastrostomy. Indications, timing and complications of the technique. *British Journal of Intensive Care* **4**, 88–92.

Powell-Tuck, J. 1978: Skin tunnel for central venous catheter – non-operative technique. *British Medical Journal* **7**, 625.

Raimundo, A.H., Rogers, J., Spiller, R.C., Grimble, G.K. and Silk, D.B.A. 1989: Effect of continuous intraduodenal enteral feeding on human colonic in-flow volumes and small bowel motility. *Gastroenterology* **404**, 96 (abstract)

Rodrigo, T.G., Kruse, J., Thill-Banarozian, M. and Carlson, R. 1989: Triple vs. single lumen central venous catheters. A prospective study in a critically ill population. *Archives of Internal Medicine* **149**, 1139–43.

Silk, D.B.A., Bray, M.J., Keele, A.M., Walters, E.R. and Duncan, H.D. 1996: Clinical evaluation of a newly designed nasogastric enteral feeding tube. *Clinical Nutrition* **15**, 285–90.

Taylor, S.J. 1988: A guide to nasogastric feeding equipment. *Professional Nurse* **3**, 91–4.

Williams, G. 1992: Hard to swallow. *Nursing Times* **88**, 63–7.

Further reading

Manning, E. and Wilkinson, D. 1996: *Peripheral parenteral nutrition techniques: the way forward. An expert guide*. Oxford: Oxford Clinical Communications.

Appendix 7.1

Guidelines for the care of patients receiving enteral feeding

Potential problem/need	Goal	Action and rationale
Presence of the nasoenteral feeding tube	The tube will remain secure, correctly positioned and patent. It will be as comfortable as possible for the patient	1. The position of the tube will be checked by aspiration of gastric contents and/or auscultation of insufflated air over the epigastrium prior to each feed and after excessive coughing or vomiting 2. The tube will be flushed with 20–50 mL sterile water before and after each intermittent feed, and if feeding is discontinued for longer than 1 h 3. The tube will be flushed with 20–50 mL sterile water before and after each enteral drug administration 4. A 20- to 50-mL syringe will be used to aspirate contents or to flush 5. Flushing will be carried out without undue force 6. The tube will be secured with tape to the nostril or the side of the face 7. Absorption of the feed will be checked after a 30-min rest by slow aspiration of gastric contents. If the residual volume is > 200 mL, continue the feed rate, and recheck after a further 4 h. If there are three consecutive residual volumes of > 200 mL, inform the medical staff

Continued . . .

Appendix 7.1 continued

Potential problem/need	Goal	Action and rationale
Insertion of the fine-bore enteral tube	The procedure will be painless and cause no trauma. Any patient who is conscious will be fully prepared for the procedure and able to co-operate where possible	1. The patient will be informed regarding the insertion technique and the purpose of the feeding tube 2. The procedure will be explained in simple terms 3. If conscious, the patient will be assisted into a semi-upright position 4. If able to do so, the patient will be asked to swallow water as the tube enters the pharynx 5. The functioning of the nasal airway will be checked 6. A signal indicating the patient's desire for the procedure to stop will be agreed upon, e.g. raising the hand 7. The tube insertion length will be gauged by (i) measuring nose to ear to xiphisternum, (ii) subtracting 50 cm from this length and (iii) dividing the result by 2 and adding 50 cm. This will ensure placement in the stomach 8. The tube will be lubricated to ensure smooth passage, and inserted using the nasal passage floor as a guide 9. If conscious, the patient will be asked to swallow as the tube enters the pharynx, and insertion will continue timed with each swallow 10. When the correct length of tube has been inserted, the tube will be lightly taped and the position checked

Presence of percutaneous endoscopic or surgical gastrostomy/jejunostomy	The tube will remain secure, correctly positioned and patent. It will be as comfortable as possible for the patient	1. Tube position will be checked after vomiting 2. The tube will be flushed with 20–50 mL of sterile water before and after each feed or drug administration 3. A 20- to 50-mL syringe will be used for flushing 4. Flushing will be carried out without undue force 5. The tube will be well secured with tape 6. The insertion site will be cleaned every 3 days, and the surrounding skin will be cleaned daily 7. The site of the gastrostomy/jejunostomy will be observed daily for leakage of gastric contents and excoriation of the surrounding skin
Potential incorrect placement or displacement of the feeding tube	Correct position of the tube will be confirmed before feeding begins	1. Gastric contents will be aspirated and tested on litmus paper which will turn pink. Litmus paper will indicate if the pH is <4 2. Bubbling of 20 mL of air will be auscultated over the epigstrium when insufflated through the feeding tube *Note:* It is still possible to hear air bubbling if the tube is in the lung (Metheny, 1990) 3. If there is any doubt about placement, i.e. if either check is not fully confirmed, then a chest X-ray will be taken
Potential xerostomia and mucosal damage (dry sore mouth)	Patient will feel comfortable and mucosa will remain intact	1. Gingiva and mucosa will be assessed for swelling, inflammation or bleeding 2. Oral care will be administered according to local policy with a minimum of twice-daily dental care using a soft toothbrush 3. A chlorhexidine mouthwash will be considered if gingivitis is evident 4. The patient's lips will be protected with petroleum jelly

Continued ...

Appendix 7.1 continued

Potential problem/need	Goal	Action and rationale
Abdominal intolerance manifested by pain, distension, bloating, nausea or vomiting	Patient will tolerate nutrition where possible, or signs of intolerance will be recognized early	1. Gastric residual volumes will be measured 4-hourly when feed is first established, and then 8-hourly. If residual volume is > 200 mL the feeding rate will not be increased but feeding will continue unless there are three consecutive volumes of > 200 mL. Alternative measures such as prokinetic agents or jejunal feeding should be considered 2. The patient's abdomen will be assessed for signs of distension 3. If distension is accompanied by abdominal pain and/or vomiting or nausea, feed will be discontinued and medical staff informed
Diarrhoea	Patient will be protected from dehydration, electrolyte imbalance and skin excoriation while the cause of diarrhoea is determined and treated	1. Potential causes will be reviewed. Alternative drugs or appropriate treatment will be prescribed. Alternative feeds (e.g. high fibre) can be reviewed with the dietitian and medical staff 2. Three consecutive stool specimens will be sent for testing for *Clostridium difficile*. If *C. difficile* is isolated, then a course of metronidazole or vancomycin will be required. Cholestyramine can be used to bind *C. difficile* toxin until antibiotic therapy is complete 3. Hypomotility agents such as loperamide or codeine phosphate may be used once enterotoxins have been ruled out *Note: DO NOT STOP FEED UNLESS DIARRHOEA REMAINS UNCONTROLLABLE DESPITE ALL OTHER INTERVENTIONS*

Constipation	The patient will continue his or her normal bowel habit	1. Records of the patient's bowel movements will be kept in the care plan or on the chart
		2. Any period longer than 3 days without bowel movement in a fed patient and 1 week in a patient not receiving feed should be noted and investigated
		3. If longer than 1 week, a *per rectum* examination should be carried out
		4. Laxatives and/or glycerin suppositories may be prescribed and further investigation carried out
Potential aspiration pneumonia	The risk of aspiration will be minimized	1. Assessment of gastric tolerance will be carried out as described above
		2. The patient will be nursed head up at a 30–45° angle
		3. The position of the tube will be checked following any violent coughing or vomiting
		4. Pulmonary secretions obtained during suctioning will be examined to ensure that no visible feed has entered the trachea
		5. If there is concern regarding aspiration, edible food colour should be added to the feed to highlight aspiration
Potential bacterial contamination	The risk from contamination will be minimized	1. Ready-to-hang or pre-mixed feed will be used wherever possible
		2. Handwashing will be carried out prior to handling feed or feeding equipment
		3. Feed will be labelled, dated and timed and will not hang for longer than 8 h
		4. Feed will not be topped up, but reservoirs will be empty prior to refilling
		5. The reservoir and giving set will be changed 24-hourly
		6. Sterile gloves will be worn when handling feed and feeding equipment for the immunocompromised patient

Continued . . .

Appendix 7.1 continued

Potential problem/need	Goal	Action and rationale
Potential hyperglycaemia	Blood glucose will remain within normal limits during feeding (4–8 mmol/L)	1. Blood glucose levels will be monitored a minimum of 4-hourly during establishment of feeding and 8-hourly once feed is established
Potential tube obstruction	The tube will remain patent	1. The tube should be flushed with 20–50 mL of sterile water (i) whenever the feed is discontinued for > 1 h, (ii) before and after any drugs given down the tube and (iii) if there is resistance to flow down the tube
		2. Crushed tablets should not be given down the tube. Discuss the possibility of dispersible or linctus forms of the drug with the pharmacy department
		3. Use continuous rather than intermittent delivery methods
Potential dehydration or fluid overload	The patient will remain in fluid balance	1. Discuss alternative feeds such as a high-calorie feed with the dietitian and medical staff if the patient is fluid restricted
		2. Review the patient's requirements for feed volumes on a daily basis

Appendix 7.2

Guidelines for the care of patient receiving parenteral feeding

Potential problem/need	Goal	Action and rationale
Enteral nutritional delivery is not possible	To meet stated nutritional requirements safely via the parenteral route	1. The prescribed amount of parenteral nutrition will be delivered over 24 h 2. Parenteral nutrition will be set up by a trained nurse according to local hospital policy 3. The procedure will be carried out under strict asepsis to avoid any potential contamination of bag, giving set or catheter 4. Ideally, the pre-mixed AIO bag will be removed from the fridge 2 h prior to use to allow it to reach room temperature 5. A volumetric intravenous infusion pump will be used to deliver the parenteral nutrition
Electrolyte imbalance	Plasma electrolyte levels will be maintained within normal limits (potassium 3.5–5.0 mmol/L, sodium 130–150 mmol/L)	1. Electrolyte levels will be monitored on a daily basis 2. There will be ECG monitoring for evidence of electrolyte-related changes 3. Electrolyte levels will be reviewed with the ICU team, dietitian and pharmacist on a daily basis

Continued . . .

Appendix 7.2 continued

Potential problem/need	Goal	Action and rationale
Potential unstable blood glucose levels	Blood glucose levels will be maintained in the range 4–10 mmol/L	1. Blood glucose levels will be measured 1- to 2-hourly when PN is first commenced and a minimum of 8-hourly once PN is established
		2. If present, medical staff will be informed if blood glucose is outside the prescribed range
		3. Intravenous insulin will be infused when necessary as per prescription to maintain blood glucose levels
		4. Infusion rates of insulin will be titrated against blood glucose levels
		5. Ideally, the insulin infusion should be discontinued 30 min prior to discontinuation of the PN
Potential phlebitis or blockage of peripheral vein during PPN	Peripheral parenteral nutrition will be delivered without blockage or phlebitis of the peripheral vein	1. The insertion site will be inspected on each shift for reddening, swelling and purulent discharge. If present, the medical staff will be informed
		2. If reddening, swelling and pain on touch (with or without purulent discharge) are present the PPN will be discontinued
		3. Prior to attachment of a new bag of PPN, and on completion of the daily volume, the peripheral cannula will be flushed
		4. A prescribed glyceryl trinitrate (GTN) patch will be placed distal to the end of the peripheral venous cannula
		5. The GTN patch will be changed every 24–48 h according to local policy

Problem	Goal	Nursing action
		6. Monitor the patient for headaches, and discontinue GTN if these occur
		7. If a ported venous cannula is used for short-term PN, it should be electively changed every 48 h
Potential catheter-related infection	Parenteral nutrition will be delivered without infection or blockage occurring as a result of inadequate management	1. Ensure only a dedicated PN lumen on a triple-lumen catheter or a tunnelled feeding line is used for delivery of PN
		2. Full aseptic precautions will be used during any manipulation of any lumen of the catheter
		3. The catheter insertion site will be inspected daily
		4. Medical staff will be informed of any reddening, swelling or purulent discharge associated with the insertion site
		5. The patient's temperature will be monitored at least twice daily, and medical staff will be informed of any pyrexia > 38°C
		6. The catheter will be flushed with heparinized saline whenever PN is disconnected for more than 10 min
Potential painful oral mucosa, gingivitis and/or xerostomia (dry mouth)	The oral mucosa will appear moist, clean, pink and free from infection or lesions	1. Oral mucosa will be inspected a minimum of once daily for signs of dryness, reddening, cracking, swelling, bleeding or infection
		2. Medical staff will be informed if there are signs of infection
		3. Mouth care will be carried out 2- to 4-hourly using a soft toothbrush and water with toothpaste twice daily
		4. The use of a chlorhexidine mouthwash will be considered if gingivitis is apparent
		5. Vaseline (petroleum jelly) will be applied to the patient's lips as required

8

Complications of enteral nutrition

The aims of this chapter are:

- to discuss the mechanical, physiological and infectious complications of enteral nutrition;
- to review the incidence, management and prevention of these problems.

Complications of enteral nutrition

Although enteral nutrition (EN) is usually considered to have fewer complications associated with its use than PN, there is still a number of potentially harmful problems that require monitoring and, where necessary, prevention. They can be grouped into mechanical, physiological and infectious categories.

Mechanical complications

These include:

- tube blockage;
- aspiration;
- nasal/pharyngeal irritation;
- tube misplacement.

Tube blockage

This can occur after discontinuation of feed, or after the administration of intermittent feed and medication. Stagnant feed or medication can congeal and linger within the tube. Repeated gastric reflux can cause feed precipitation.

The following measures have helped to eliminate this problem almost completely.

1. Wherever possible, avoid administering crushed tablets down the enteral tube. Any drugs used should be either soluble or in the form of an elixir.
2. The enteral tube should be flushed with 20–50 mL of sterile water before and after each feed and following the administration of medication.
3. Use a polyurethane or PVC material tube with the largest possible internal diameter.

Aspiration

Pulmonary aspiration is a major potential complication of enteral nutrition in the critically ill patient. The incidence of aspiration in critically ill patients has been reported to be up to 40 per cent of patients who are orally or tube fed (Berger and Adams, 1989).

Critically ill patients often have more than one risk factor that increases the risk of aspiration. These are, (i) depressed level of consciousness, (ii) decreased rate of gastric emptying, (iii) the presence of a nasogastric/tracheal tube (Sands, 1991).

The following factors predispose the patient to pulmonary aspiration:

- depressed level of consciousness;
- drugs (CNS depressants);
- alcohol;
- epilepsy;
- coma;
- tracheal intubation;
- nasogastric intubation;
- gastro-oesophageal dysfunction, e.g. vomiting, regurgitation;
- gastric distension;
- gastro-oesophageal reflux;
- decreased oesophageal motility;
- flat or head-down positioning.

Endotracheal tube cuff design and cuff status can influence the incidence of aspiration (Adam and Osborne, 1997; Elpern *et al.*, 1987). Intubated patients can aspirate gastric contents despite an inflated cuff.

The risk of aspiration can be reduced by the following measures:

- a small-bore feeding tube – aspiration is still possible, but the oesophageal sphincter is less compromised by the smaller diameter of the tube;
- ensuring proper tube placement prior to commencing each feed and following vomiting or regurgitation of feed:

   monitor the tube position by initially marking the tube on its external surface and checking that this has not migrated outwards;

   monitor the tube position internally by performing gastric aspiration and a chest X-ray;
- positioning the patient upright (45°) during feeding and 1 h post feeding providing that the patient's cardiovascular status allows this;
- checking for abdominal distension. If distension is present, check gastric residual volume. If this is > 200 mL, stop the feed and inform senior medical staff;
- checking gastric residual volumes at 4-hourly intervals for the first 24 h of feeding and if there are signs of abdominal intolerance. If feed is tolerated, volumes can be checked at 8-hourly intervals;
- discontinuing feed for 1 h prior to any 'head-down' procedures, such as insertion of central venous lines.

Nasal/pharyngeal irritation

Selection of the correct tube size is essential. Large-bore nasogastric tubes, e.g. Ryle's tubes, may reduce the competency of the oesophageal sphincter, thus increasing the risk of reflux and aspiration.

Due to their size and the type of material used, Ryle's tubes have been associated with patient discomfort, oesophagitis, pharyngitis, tracheal fistula formation and rupture of oesophageal varices. They can interfere with coughing and spontaneous respiration (Cataldi-Betcher *et al.*, 1983; Taylor, 1988; Fawcett and Yeoman, 1991).

Preventive measures:

- use a fine-bore feeding tube;
- administer nasal and oral care 2-hourly.

Tube displacement

This can occur with any strenuous coughing or retching. In general, patients undergoing continuous feeding should have the tube position checked by aspiration and pH testing and/or insufflation of air following any vigorous coughing or retching. The tube should be secured firmly to the face or nose, and loosely secured to the pillow to prevent direct traction on the tube.

Physiological complications

Diarrhoea

Diarrhoea is a frequent complication of all gastrointestinal disturbances (Cataldi-Betcher *et al.*, 1983) and has been found to develop in 10 to 25 per cent of enterally fed patients (Berger and Adams, 1989).

However, in the critically ill patient the causes of diarrhoea are often multifactorial.

Causes of diarrhoea have changed over the years. The emphasis has moved from the deleterious effects of hypertonic feeds and bolus feed administration to the side-effects of other drugs and bacterial contamination. Drugs that have been particularly associated with causing diarrhoea include:

- antibiotics;
- magnesium-containing antacids;
- electrolyte elixirs;
- digoxin;
- methyl-dopa;
- laxatives.

Therefore, if diarrhoea becomes a problem, one of the first interventions should be review of the prescription chart and alteration or discontinuation of any drugs that are known to cause diarrhoea.

It may be useful to administer antidiarrhoeal drugs, e.g. loperamide, diphenoxylate hydrochloride and codeine phosphate, if it is known that the diarrhoea is drug-related. For antimicrobial-induced diarrhoea, pectin and cholestyramine may be preferred (Berger and Adams, 1989).

Rapid infusion rates and bolus feeding increase the incidence of diarrhoea (Cataldi-Belcher *et al.*, 1983; Williams, 1992), whereas the use of a continuous pump infusion minimizes the incidence of diarrhoea.

Lactose intolerance, together with high osmolarity and high-fat-content feeds have been cited as a potential cause of diarrhoea in the past. However, commercially prepared feeds no longer contain lactose, and the majority are no longer hyperosmolar.

Hypoalbuminaemia

This may cause osmotic diarrhoea if it is associated with a low capillary osmotic pressure (COP).

The administration of artificial colloids can maintain an adequate COP despite hypoalbuminaemia. However, if the COP is reduced with hypoalbuminaemia, the feed within the intestinal lumen may create an osmotic gradient with fluid moving into rather than out of the intestine, thus causing a loose watery stool (Adam and Osborne, 1997).

1. Consider potential causes of diarrhoea.
2. Chart the frequency, colour and amount of diarrhoea.
3. If more than 3 loose watery stools are passed per day, send a specimen for MC&S. (Note: Do NOT stop feed unless in association with a severe absorptive disorder or an infection, such as *Clostridium difficile*).

Nausea and vomiting

Nausea and vomiting can occur in 5 to 20 per cent of cases (Payne-James *et al.*, 1988; Berger and Adams, 1989). The causes are varied and include gastric reflux, gastric hypomotility, gastrointestinal dysfunction or, occasionally, fat intolerance.

Metaclopramide, cisapride and erythromycin can be used to treat delayed gastric emptying.

Preventative measures include the following:

1. checking for residual volumes (stop feed if residual volume is > 200 mL);
2. maintaining the patient at a 45° angle during feeding, although this can be impractical, if not impossible, in some critically ill patients;
3. use of prokinetic agents, e.g. metaclopromide, erythromycin, cisapride;
4. use of naso/jejunal/duodenal feeding tubes.

Hyperglycaemia

Increased blood glucose levels during enteral nutrition can result in patients who:

- are unable to respond to the increased glucose load by increasing insulin production;
- exhibit 'insulin resistance' and have continued hepatic gluconeogenesis despite adequate glucose ingestion and blood glucose levels;
- are insulin-dependent and non-insulin-dependent diabetics.

Assiduous blood glucose monitoring ensures early recognition of the problem, and the institution of insulin infusions titrated to maintain normal blood glucose levels may be necessary.

Hypercapnia

Excess carbohydrate calories may induce increased carbon dioxide production. Patients who are unable to increase their respiratory performance sufficiently to excrete the added carbon dioxide load may develop acute hypercapnic respiratory failure as a result. This may affect the weaning of patients.

Mechanism of excess carbohydrate carbon dioxide production

Excess carbohydrate ingestion will result in lipogenesis (fat production) through the hepatic route. The production of free fatty acids results in a high volume of carbon dioxide production – for each calorie of glucose converted to fat, 3 mL of carbon dioxide must be expired.

Electrolyte/trace element imbalance

Electrolytes

Careful monitoring of electrolyte levels is essential. The frequency of monitoring should be 4 to 6-hourly when feeding is first commenced, and as indicated in Table 8.1 once feeding is established.

> **Box 8.1** Normal plasma electrolyte levels
>
> | | |
> |---|---|
> | Sodium | 135–150 mmol/L |
> | Potassium | 3.5–5.0 mmol/L |
> | Magnesium | 0.5–1.1 mmol/L |
> | Calcium | 2.25–2.65 mmol/L |
> | Phosphate | 0.8–1.4 mmol/L |

Critically ill patients can experience considerable variations in intracellular and extracellular electrolyte levels, with severely deleterious effects. The causes of electrolyte variations include:

- increased urinary loss following cellular catabolism and loss of intracellular mass (potassium, phosphate);
- increased serum aldosterone levels (potassium loss and sodium retention);
- acute stress response and increased ADH secretion (sodium retention);
- alterations in cellular permeability (potassium, sodium);
- nutritional replacement following malnutrition (phosphate, potassium, magnesium) (see refeeding syndrome);
- metabolic acidosis and alkalosis (potassium, bicarbonate, chloride, sodium);
- gastrointestinal tract losses and diarrhoea (potassium, sodium, magnesium);
- concurrent administration of amphotericin (potassium loss);
- low serum albumin levels (calcium).

Trace elements

The majority of plasma trace element levels are not reliable as an indicator of trace element deficiency, and thus diagnosis can be difficult. Trace elements are hugely important in a range of bodily functions (see Chapter 2), and deficiencies are associated with impaired immune function, wound healing, glucose tolerance and platelet aggregation.

While preconstituted feeding regimes all contain the recommended daily levels of electrolytes, vitamins, minerals and trace elements, these are based on the requirements of healthy individuals and may be seriously disturbed in the critically ill. Electrolytes should be adjusted on the basis of need, and trace elements and minerals should be based on clinical judgement.

Table 8.1 Monitoring nutritional support in the critically ill patient

Variable	Monitoring frequency
Electrolytes	Daily
Serum magnesium, calcium and phosphate	Twice weekly
Acid-base status	Daily
Gastric residuals (aspirate)	Four-hourly when starting feeding; 8-hourly when established
Abdominal function (distension, vomiting, nausea, diarrhoea, constipation)	Continuously
Flow rate and volume infused	Hourly
Blood glucose	Eight-hourly
Urinalysis for glucose and ketones	Daily
Urea and creatinine (plasma)	Daily
Urea and creatinine clearance (urinary)	24-h urine collection weekly
Fluid balance	Accurate hourly records
Weight (if mobile or on a weigh bed)	For fluid status, daily; for nutritional status, weekly
Haematological and coagulation screens	Every 1–2 days
Serum albumin, proteins, liver function tests (LFTs)	Weekly
Trace elements such as copper, zinc, etc.	As required

Fluid overload

Patients who are unable to tolerate high fluid volumes due to cardiac or renal failure, and also in severe acute respiratory distress syndrome (ARDS), may receive excess fluid loads from their nutritional regimens. Care should be taken to ensure that the administration of enteral nutrition is not in excess of the fluid volume which the patient can tolerate. High-energy enteral feeds (1.5–2 kcal/mL) should be substituted to ensure that the patient receives as many as possible of his or her nutrient requirements.

Infectious complications

Critically ill patients as a group are highly vulnerable to infection. Factors which increase the risk include:

- endotracheal intubation;
- invasive venous access and monitoring;
- suppression of immunological response as a result of disease, sepsis or stress;
- urinary catheterization;
- trauma and wounds;
- environmental risks of cross-contamination from other critically ill patients.

Both methods of nutritional support carry increased infection risks, but there is evidence to suggest an increased incidence of infectious complications associated with parenteral nutrition (Peterson *et al.*, 1988; Kudsk *et al.*, 1992; Moore *et al.*, 1995). The contributing factors are:

- intravenous access allowing bacterial contamination directly into the venous circulation;
- reduced integrity of the gut barrier due to loss of luminal nutrients, etc. (see Chapter 4);
- suppression of local, systemic and lung immune responses to bacterial challenge (reported in PN-fed animal studies, although this evidence is not supported in humans yet) (Lin *et al.*, 1996);
- increased incidence of uncontrolled hyperglycaemia associated with increased risk of infection (Pomposelli and Bistrian, 1994).

The risks of infection from parenteral nutrition are more likely to be life-threatening than those associated with enteral nutrition. However, both forms of nutritional support are associated with infection as a result of bacterial contamination.

Box 8.2

Infection risks associated with enteral nutrition
Infective diarrhoea – incidence 11% (Belknap *et al.*, 1990)
Pulmonary aspiration/ nosocomial pneumonia – incidence 12% (Kudsk *et al.*, 1992)

Infection risks associated with parenteral nutrition
Bacteraemia – incidence 9.1% (Ioannides-Demos *et al.*, 1995)
Catheter-related sepsis – incidence 13.3% (Kudsk *et al.*, 1992)

Bacterial contamination

It is now well recognized that enteral feeds may become contaminated with micro-organisms during the preparation and administration of an enteral feed (Anderton, 1993).

The design of the administration systems make it impossible to clean them effectively. Bacteria and food residue may remain after washing, and therefore provide a medium for bacteria when the system is refilled with sterile feed.

It is *not* advisable to clean and disinfect the equipment in preparation for another use. Administration equipment should be for single use only. If infection does occur, then the potential source of bacterial contamination should be thoroughly investigated. If diarrhoea is a resulting problem, then a sample must be sent for culture.

Preventive measures should include the following:

- use a clean procedure in the preparation and administration of feed;
- change the giving set and reservoirs every 24 h;
- do not top up feed;
- feed should not be left hanging in reservoirs for more than 8 h.

Complications of gastrostomy and jejunostomy feeding

Complications of percutaneous endoscopic gastrostomy can be divided into major and minor categories. Major complications are defined as those requiring celiotomy, or which result in death or prolonged hospitalization.

Major complications of Gauderer Ponsky and Russell PEGs range from 0 to 4.4 per cent, whilst minor complications occur in 4 to 16 per cent of patients (Miller *et al.*, 1989; Peters and Westaby, 1994).

Complications associated with tube and/or feed delivery include:

- pulmonary aspiration;
- tube displacement;
- pneumoperitoneum;
- gastrocolic fistula;
- haemorrhage.

Infectious complications include:

- peristomal wound infection;
- necrotizing fasciitis;
- peritonitis.

Complications associated with tube and/or feed delivery

Pulmonary aspiration

Pulmonary aspiration can occur at any point during the insertion of the tube, or at any point afterwards as a consequence of feeding. It occurs in 0.7 per cent – 1.6 per cent of patients (Peters and Westaby, 1994).

Regurgitation and aspiration of feed are more likely to occur in elderly, debilitated patients and those with poor gag reflexes or neuromotor swallowing disorders (Silk, 1987). The presence of an endotracheal tube is also significantly more likely to be associated with regurgitation of feed, although the presence of an endotracheal cuff offers some protection from large-volume aspiration, e.g. during vomiting (Dotson *et al.* 1994).

The following measures are used to prevent aspiration:

- Insertion should be performed quickly.
- Ensure that proper tube placement takes place and check the position prior to commencing each feed, regularly (minimum of 8-hourly) where feeding is continuous and following any vigorous coughing or retching.
- The patient's upper body should be raised to approximately 30–45° from the horizontal to decrease the likelihood of regurgitation.
- Regular (minimum of 8-hourly) aspiration of gastric contents should take place, or aspiration prior to feeds if bolus feeding is taking place. If more than 200 mL of feed are aspirated, then the feeding rate should continued and further aspiration carried out at 4-hourly intervals.

Pneumoperitoneum

This is the presence of free air in the abdominal cavity. Benign pneumoperitoneum is a commonly reported complication of PEG placement and occurs in 21–38 per cent of patients (Mamel, 1989; Peters and Westaby, 1994). It generally has no clinical significance, and tends to occur as a result of over-insufflation of the stomach.

When a pneumoperitoneum is suspected, Gastrografin screening will confirm the diagnosis.

Massive pneumoperitoneum can occur in ventilated patients in whom tracheo-oesophageal fistulae have developed, resulting in the transmission of ventilator pressure to the gastrointestinal tract (Peters and Westaby, 1994).

Haemorrhage

This is an uncommon complication which occurs in 0–2.5 per cent of cases (Fawcett and Yeoman, 1991).

It occurs as a result of abnormal clotting, pressure necrosis, or abrasion of gastric mucosa, or it may be secondary to gastric ulcers which appear at the site of insertion due to excessive traction from the PEG.

This complication presents as pain, haematemesis, melaena and evidence of blood in the gastrostomy tube. Diagnosis is made by endoscopy and exclusion of other causes of bleeding.

The gastrostomy tube tension should be decreased and a course of H_2 antagonists or proton-pump inhibitors prescribed (Peters and Westaby, 1994).

Gastrocolic fistula

Occurring as a rare complication due to accidental insertion of the tube through the stomach wall, the gastrocolic fistula forms a passage between stomach and bowel. A skilled technician and rigorous insertion technique will reduce the likelihood of this complication.

In general, the fistula will close spontaneously once the PEG is removed.

Infectious complications

Peristomal wound infection

This is the most common complication associated with PEG insertion, occurring in 5–30 per cent of patients (Mamel, 1989). However, the use of prophylactic antibiotics prior to insertion has significantly reduced this incidence.

Peristomal wound infection can be fatal, so prompt treatment is required. In the first instance, the tube tension should be checked and frequent site dressings carried out. Prolonged and persistent pain should not be considered normal after 2–3 days.

Necrotizing fasciitis

This is an uncommon soft tissue infection which can result from a peristomal wound infection if this is not recognized early enough. Treatment is by surgical debridement and the administration of broad-spectrum antibiotics.

Peritonitis and tube displacement

The incidence is reported to be between 0 and 1.2 per cent of PEG patients. The commonest cause of peritonitis is the premature removal of the PEG tube before a fibrous tract can be formed between the gastric and abdominal walls. This may occur as a result of mishandling of the tube by a patient, or it may be due to the deflation or rupture of the balloon, causing the stomach to move away from the abdominal wall. Tubes may erode through the gastric wall if excessive tension is present.

The following measures are used to prevent peritonitis.

- Ensure that the tube is well secured by tape and/or dressing to prevent dislodgement.
- Check the tension of the outer abdominal bumper/disc to ensure that the correct tension is applied as soon after insertion as is possible.
- Check the tension of the tube at each dressing change to ensure that it has not increased.

References

Adam, S.K. and Batson, S. 1997: A study of problems associated with the delivery of enteral feed in the critically ill in 5 intensive care units in the UK. *Intensive Care Medicine* **23**, 261–6.

Adam, S.K. and Osborne, S. 1977: *Critical care nursing: science and practice*. Oxford: Oxford University Press.

Anderton, A.L. 1993: Bacterial contamination of enteral feeds and feeding systems. *Clinical Nutrition* **12**, S16–S32.

Belknap, D.C., Davidson, L.J. and Flournoy, D.J. 1990: Microorganisms and diarrhea in enterally fed intensive care unit patients. *Journal of Parenteral and Enteral Nutrition* **14**, 622–8.

Berger, R. and Adams, L. 1989: Nutritional support in the critical care setting. Part 2. *Chest* **96**, 372–80.

Cataldi-Betcher, E.L., Seltzer, M.H., Slocum, B.A. and Jones, K.W. 1983: Complications occurring during enteral nutrition support. A prospective study. *Journal of Parenteral and Enteral Nutrition* **7**, 546–52.

Dotson, R.G., Robinson, R.G. and Pingleton, S.K. 1994: Gastro-esophageal reflux with nasogastric tubes: effect of tube sizes. *American Journal of Respiratory and Critical Care Medicine* **149**, 1659–62.

Elpern, E.H., Jacobs, E.R. and Bone, R.C. 1987: Incidence of aspiration in tracheally intubated adults. *Heart and Lung* **16**, 527–31.

Fawcett, H. and Yeoman, C. 1991: A tube to suit all nasogastric needs? *Professional Nurse* **6**, 324–9.

Ioannides-Demos, L.L., Liolios, L., Topliss, D.J. and Mclean, A.J. 1995: A prospective audit of total parenteral nutrition at a major teaching hospital. *Medical Journal of Australia* **163**, 233–7.

Kelly, K. Lewis, B., Gentile, D., Benjamin, E., Waye, J. and Iberti, T. 1988: Use of percutaneous gastrostomy in the intensive care patient. *Critical Care Medicine* **16**, 62–3.

Kudsk, K.A., Croce, M.A., Fabian, T.C. *et al.* 1992: Enteral versus parenteral feeding. Effects on septic morbidity after blunt and penetrating abdominal trauma. *Annals of Surgery* **215**, 503–11.

Lin, M.T., Saito, H., Fukushima, R. *et al.* 1996: Route of nutritional supply influences local, systemic and remote organ responses to intraperitoneal bacterial challenge. *Annals of Surgery* **223**, 84–93.

Maki, D.G. and Will, L. 1984: Colonization and infection associated with transparent dressings for central venous, arterial and Hickmann catheters: a comparative trial. In: Program and Abstracts of the 24th Interscience Conference on Antimicrobial Agents and Chemotherapy.

Maki, D.G., Stolz, S. and Wheeler, S. 1991: A prospective random-ized, three-way clinical comparison of a novel, highly permeable, polyurethane dressing with 206 Swan-Ganz pulmonary artery catheters: opsite IV 3000 versus Tegaderm versus gauze and tape. I Cutaneous colonization under the dressing, catheter-related infection. In: Maki, D.G. (ed.). *Improving catheter site care*. London and New York: Royal Society of Medicine Services Ltd, International Congress & Symposium Series, No. 179, 61–6.

Mamel, J.J. 1989: Percutaneous endoscopic gastrostomy. *American Journal of Gastroenterology* **85**, 703–10.

Miller, R.E., Castlemain, B., Laacqua, F.J. and Kotler, D.P. 1989: Percutaneous endoscopic gastrostomy. Results in 316 patients and review of literature. *Surgical Endoscopy* **3**, 186–90.

Moore, F.A., Moore, E.E. and Haenel, J.B. 1995: Clinical benefits of early postinjury feeding. *Clinical Intensive Care* **6**, 21–7.

Payne-James, J., Rees, R., Grimble, G. and Silk, D. 1988: Enteral nutrition: clinical applications. *Intensive Therapy and Clinical Monitoring* **11**, 239–46.

Peters, R.A. and Westaby, D. 1994: Percutaneous endoscopic gastrostomy: indications, timing and complications of the technique. *British Journal of Intensive Care* **4**, 88–92.

Peterson, V.M., Moore, E.E., Jones, T.N. *et al.* 1988: Total enteral nutrition versus total parenteral nutrition after major torso injury: attenuation of hepatic protein reprioritisation. *Surgery* **104**, 199–207.

Pomposelli, J.J. and Bistrian, B.R. 1994: Is total parenteral nutrition immunosuppressive? *New Horizons* **2**, 224–9.

Sands, J. 1991: Incidence of pulmonary aspiration in intubated patients receiving enteral nutrition through wide and narrow bore nasogastric feeding tubes. *Heart and Lung* **20**, 75–80.

Silk, D. 1987: Towards the optimization of enteral nutrition. *Clinical Nutrition* **6**, 61–74.

Taylor, S.J. 1988: A guide to nasogastric feeding equipment. *Professional Nurse* **3**, 91–4.

Williams, G. 1992: Hard to swallow. *Nursing Times* **88**, 63–7.

Air embolism

This is potentially a problem during insertion. The risk is significantly reduced by positioning the patient into a 20° or 30° head-down tilt position prior to venepuncture, thus raising the intrathoracic and central venous pressure.

Catheter misplacement

This can often occur during catheter insertion of the subclavian vein. Misplacement occurs more frequently on the right side because of the sudden descent of the superior vena cava from the point of junction of the right subclavian vein (Berger and Adams, 1989). A chest X-ray should be carried out either during or immediately post-insertion in order to detect this complication.

Catheter misplacement with perforation of a vessel or the advancement of the catheter into the pleural space, mediastinum or pericardium can result in dangerous complications of haematoma, haemopneumothorax, upper airway obstruction or pericardial tamponade.

Haematoma

This can occur as the result of trauma to the vein or its surrounding tissues on insertion.

Subclavian artery puncture

This is another potential problem, particularly during subclavian vein catheterization. If subclavian artery puncture occurs, the needle should be withdrawn and pressure applied over the artery for approximately 5 min. Catheterization on the next occasion should occur approximately 1 cm lower than the original needle insertion.

Arrhythmias

These can occur during catheter insertion, usually because of the close proximity of the catheter tip to the sino-atrial node. If any arrhythmias occur, immediate withdrawal of the catheter tip to a position in the superior vena cava will rectify the situation (Grimble *et al.*, 1989).

Cardiac tamponade

This is a rare complication that results from perforation of the vessel wall by the catheter or introducing wire. It is becoming rarer in incidence due to the use of silicone and polyurethane catheters which are much softer and more pliable to manipulate. The use of flexible-tip guide wires is now less likely to cause this complication.

Treatment of the complication is urgent. If the catheter remains *in situ*, the lowering of the infusion bag may allow for some retrograde flow of blood or PN from the pericardial cavity. If there is no catheter *in situ*, urgent pericardiocentesis will be required.

Central catheter-related complications

Complications that occur after catheter insertion can be minimized by strict adherence to policies and protocols of care.

The main central catheter related complications are:

- infection;
- occlusion;
- air embolism;
- central venous thrombosis.

Infection

The administration of PN is of paramount importance, and in many cases, it is the patient's only source of nutrients and fluid. Any violation of accepted policies or protocols could have serious consequences for the patient, particularly if infection occurs. Strict asepsis is mandatory during any procedure which involves breaking a closed system.

The portals of bacterial entry are:

- the catheter entry/exit site;
- administration sets;
- parenteral nutrition fluid;
- the hub of the catheter.

Catheter entry/exit site

The catheter forms a direct link between the skin surface and the venous circulation. It is imperative that regular dressing changes are carried out in order to disinfect the area, reduce the skin flora and inhibit the colonization of bacteria. The type of dressing, together with the proposed duration of the dressing, influences the incidence of infection.

Transparent film dressings

Transparent film dressings have some advantages over gauze dressings and have improved over the years. Initially, transparent dressings – although useful in facilitating easy visual inspection – were prone to moisture accumulation due to the increased surface humidity and skin flora colonization which was shown in some cases to increase infection (Powell *et al.*, 1982; Maki and Will, 1984). However, the introduction of improved moisture-responsive dressings, e.g. IV 3000, has significantly reduced the incidence of infection by preventing moisture accumulation. Thus the stability and duration of the dressing are enhanced (Maki *et al.*, 1991), and the dressing can be left *in situ* for up to 5 days. Regular visual site inspections should be undertaken and the dressing changed if there is a loss of integrity, contamination, or an accumulation of blood or serous fluid.

Occlusive dressings

Occlusive dressings, e.g. Melonin (Smith & Nephew) or Mepore (Mölnlycke), are effective for tunnelled feeding catheters. They should be renewed twice weekly or if damaged or uncomfortable (Stotter *et al.*, 1987; De Ciccio *et al.*, 1989). Untunnelled catheters should be redressed every 48 h unless transparent film dressings are being used, as the catheter itself has no mechanical barrier. Microorganisms can therefore enter the venous circulation with greater ease.

Observation of the site should be undertaken daily for any redness, discharge of pus or exudate, soreness or swelling. Complete or incomplete anchorage of the catheter should be noted. Infection of the catheter tunnel, itself a complication of an exit site infection, is characterized by pain and redness. This complication does not respond well to treatment and is therefore an indication for catheter removal.

Administration sets

The incorrect use of administration sets and additional luer-lock connections can pose a threat. Changing the administration set daily, together with the wearing of sterile gloves and the use of chlorhexidine (0.5 per cent in 70 per cent spirit) to clean connections should eliminate infection from this route. However, the use of intravenous filters placed between the cannula and the administration set may be helpful in preventing bacteria from gaining access to the vein, as well as preventing infusion of certain particulates (Murphy and Lipman, 1987; Johnson, 1994).

Parenteral nutrition fluid

Contamination of infusion fluids is rarely a problem now, due to enhanced quality control and strict manufacturing recommendations. Two- or three-litre PN bags are usually compounded in designated sterile production units. However, PN solutions manufactured in bottles and sold for storage and subsequent mixing in a ward environment can pose a threat if knowledge and policy adherence are poor. Furthermore, it is essential that no additions of either drug or nutrient should be made to any bag or bottle at ward level. If additional drugs or nutrients are required, then the solution must be returned to pharmacy in order to reduce the risk of contamination and incompatibility. All solutions should be stored at 4°C in a designated PN refrigerator to prevent micro-organism growth and maintain stability. PN solutions should be used within the stated time limit (Murphy and Lipman, 1987).

Hub of catheter

Many studies have been undertaken over the years to assess the infection risk of the catheter hub. Catheter-related sepsis appears to originate from a catheter-tip infection which has migrated from an infected hub (Sitges-Serra *et al.*, 1984a). Follow-up studies have confirmed that hub colonization by micro-organisms is the common point of entry (Sitges-Serra *et al.*, 1984a, b; Linares *et al.*, 1985; Stotter *et al.*, 1987). Nursing care must therefore ensure that manipulation of the hub is kept to a minimum. It should be thoroughly cleaned at each dressing change, and covered with the appropriate dressing as dictated by local policy.

Catheter-related sepsis (CRS)

This is defined as a clinical episode of systemic illness with isolation of an identical organism from both catheter tip and peripheral blood in the absence of any obvious primary infective source (Kohlhart *et al.*, 1994). CRS continues to be a serious and constant threat to patients receiving PN, and is a potentially lethal complication which is associated with increased morbidity, increased cost, and in some cases increased mortality (Freund and Rimon, 1990). The incidence of CRS can be significantly reduced if the following points are adhered to.

1. Central venous catheters are inserted by the same experienced operator, either a doctor or a nutrition nurse specialist, in a strict sterile environment.
2. Catheters are tunnelled subcutaneously.
3. Catheter entry and exit sites are dressed by a small number of experienced nurses who are familiar with the hospital PN policy.
4. Infusion solutions and administration sets are changed by experienced nurses who are familiar with the hospital PN policy.
5. Infusion solutions are compounded by experienced pharmacy staff inside a laminar-flow biological safety cabinet, or in the production unit of the hospital pharmacy. If these facilities are not available, then reputable commercial solutions should be used.
6. No additions are made to the infusion solution outside the pharmacy.
7. The central venous feeding line, i.e. the dedicated single-lumen catheter or the dedicated lumen of a multilumen catheter, is used exclusively for PN.

Diagnosis of CRS

Patients receiving PN often suffer from infections at sites other than that of the central venous catheter. This may be due to their underlying disease, together with the complications associated with it. Diagnosis of CRS is usually based on clinical evidence. Infection can be either localized or systemic (Elliott *et al.*, 1994).

Clinical evidence of infection includes:

- oedema;
- erythema;
- thrombophlebitis;
- exudate formate;
- pain at insertion site;
- pyrexia.

Systemic infections associated with the catheter are not always easy to diagnose. A low-grade pyrexia may be present with no obvious cause, together with no response to the administration of broad-spectrum antibiotics.

Most data suggest that virtually all catheter-related infections and instances of CRS are caused by *Staphylococcus epidermidis* (coagulase-negative Staphylococci) and *Staphylococcus aureus* (Norwood *et al.*, 1991; Roberts, 1993). Both pathogens are thought to originate from the skin and then migrate to different catheter segments (Sitges-Serra *et al.*, 1984; Linares *et al.*, 1985; Norwood *et al* 1991). *Staphylococcus epidermidis* has been found to be more adherent to the surface of plastic catheters than other organisms. The organism may stay in place indefinitely, and has been found to develop microcolonies which produce a heavy colonization after 12 h. These separate colonies produce a slime coating which adheres to the catheter and protects it from antibiotics and other types of infection. It would seem feasible, therefore, that with poor manipulation and inadequate care of the catheter and the entry/exit site, the organism could be transferred back and forth from catheter to skin, thus causing further infection (Norwood *et al.*, 1991; Roberts, 1993).

Treatment of CRS

If catheter-related sepsis is suspected, an urgent nursing and medical assessment is essential, including inspection of the entry/exit site. It is important that other possible sources of infection are excluded before it is assumed to be catheter related. Specimens of sputum, urine and wound swabs should be sent to bacteriology as appropriate. If no other cause for the sepsis is found, then ideally the catheter should be removed and the tip sent for culture. However, this is not always feasible, particularly in the ICU environment. In the first instance, a physical examination by a member of the medical staff should be undertaken and central and peripheral blood cultures obtained. Whilst waiting for the results of these cultures, it may be advisable to stop PN and seal the catheter with a heparin lock, together with the administration of antibiotics, although this will depend on local policy (Pennington, 1996). If the temperature subsides, it is probable that the catheter is the source of infection. It should be removed and the catheter tip sent for culture, with a pre-moistened swab taken from the entry/exit site. However, in many intensive-care units replacing a catheter over a guide wire is considered to be an alternative to complete withdrawal from a site. This method may be useful for diagnosing CRS, and less traumatic for the patient (Roberts, 1993). However, one criticism of this method is that organisms may in the process be transferred either to the site or to the new catheter (Norwood *et al.*, 1991). If the pyrexia persists, then some other cause for the sepsis should be sought. If the results of the investigations indicate that the catheter is not the source of infection, then PN can be continued and the infection treated appropriately.

Occlusion

The main causes of occlusion are:

- clotting;
- malpositioning;
- kinking;
- accumulation of lipid or calcium deposits;
- formation of a fibrin sleeve around the catheter.

Other influencing factors also have a role. These include:

- the type and size of catheter;
- the duration of catheter placement;
- the skill of the person performing a flush or lock procedure;
- the type of solutions infused into the catheter (Cottee, 1995).

Clotting

Clotting can be due to the type of catheter material (Cottee, 1995). Polyurethane is much preferred to polyvinylchloride (PVC). The former has a smoother surface, which is known to reduce the incidence of platelet adherence, phlebitis and subsequent infection. Hydromer-coated polyurethane catheters have recently been shown to reduce thrombus formation, fibrin deposition and platelet adhesion even further.

The prevention of occlusion can be aided by adopting the following measures.

1. Administer Hepsal or saline to maintain patency when parenteral nutrition is not being infused.

2. The time period between stopping and recommencing feed should be no longer than 1 h in order to prevent clotting within the catheter.

3. An infusion pump should always be used. If one is not available for any reason, then the clamps and devices for controlling the infusion rate should be frequently checked and adjusted to maintain the flow.

4. Administration sets should be checked regularly and positioned to avoid kinking of either the set or the catheter itself.

5. When the administration set is changed, the time period between disconnection of the old set and connection of the new set to the catheter should be kept to a minimum.

If the infusion has stopped and no reason for the occlusion can be found, then a chest X-ray should be taken to provide confirmation. The British Association of Parenteral and Enteral Nutrition (BAPEN) suggests that the line should be flushed with 10 mL of 20 per cent ethanol solution before the application of a heparin lock. Ethanol locks can help to free lines that have been partially occluded by the laying down of lipid deposits. However, if this is not successful, then the administration of 5000 units of urokinase can be used to clear the catheter, particularly if there is evidence of fibrin occlusion. Great care must be taken in the intensive-care unit because of the increased risk of bleeding.

Air embolism

Air must not be allowed to enter the catheter when it is either disconnected from or reconnected to the administration set, due to the risk of air embolus. To reduce this risk, the following precautions should be taken.

1. Connections on all equipment, i.e. catheter, administration set and extension line, should have luer-lock devices in order to prevent accidental disconnection of the infusion system.

2. During changes of the administration set, the catheter should be clamped using suitable clamps. If it is not possible to clamp the catheter, then the 20°–30°C head-down tilt position should be adopted and the patient, if able, instructed to perform the Valsalva manoeuvre (in which he or she is asked to breathe in and try to force the air out with the mouth tightly closed).

Central venous thrombosis (CVT)

Thrombosis of a central vein (usually a subclavian vein) is a rare complication. If it occurs, then it tends to develop a few weeks after insertion.

The symptoms of central venous thrombosis are:

- pyrexia;
- pulmonary embolism;
- subclavian vein thrombosis;
- occlusion of the superior vena cava with facial swelling (Pennington, 1996).

It is more likely to occur in patients with a decreased thromboplastin time or with low levels of antithrombin III (Berger and Adams, 1989). Diagnosis is confirmed by bilateral upper limb venography.

The incidence of CVT can be influenced by:

- the type of catheter material – there is an increased risk of CVT when PVC catheters are used, and a reduced risk if hydromer-coated polyurethane catheters are used;
- the use of heparin infusion/flush to minimize fibrin sleeve formation;
- volume depletion;
- any physical factor which may hinder blood flow;
- thrombogenic stimuli, including infection.

Treatment

1. Administer streptokinase infusion for 48 h to restore patency, or as directed by local policy.
2. Administer heparin, as directed by local policy.
3. Thereafter, administer warfarin.

Metabolic complications in parenteral nutrition

Hyperglycaemia

As with enteral nutrition, increases in blood glucose level can occur as a result of parenteral nutrition. The problem is much more frequent, and is more likely to require insulin to control it.

Table 9.2 Typical sliding scale for insulin

Blood glucose (mmol/L)	Insulin infusion rate (units/h)
> 20	4
15–20	2
10–15	1
7.5–10	0
0–7.5	0

Assiduous blood glucose-monitoring ensures early recognition of the problem, and either insulin infusions or a sliding scale of insulin administration (Table 9.2) can be used to control blood glucose levels.

Monitoring blood glucose during parenteral nutrition

Blood glucose-monitoring should occur every 15 to 30 min following initial commencement of PN, until blood glucose levels stabilize. Krzywda *et al*. (1993) found that the blood glucose response to PN is rapid and almost complete within 60 mins. Insulin infusions are necessary in many critically ill patients, and will require titration to maintain goals. It is unnecessary to start regimens at a reduced rate and work up to the nutritional goal, provided that blood glucose-monitoring is carried out.

Hypoglycaemia

A sudden drop in blood glucose can be associated with abrupt discontinuation of parenteral nutrition. If the patient is receiving insulin, then there should not be any interruption in the delivery of PN. However, if this is unavoidable, then insulin should be discontinued at least 30 min prior to the end of the feed.

Refeeding syndrome

This is a term used to describe a collection of phenomena, including severe hypophosphataemia, hypomagnesaemia, hypokalaemia and other metabolic complications seen in malnourished patients who are receiving concentrated calories via total parenteral nutrition following a period of malnutrition.

Severe hypophosphataemia and other electrolyte disturbances have been described in the past in critically ill patients (Tovey *et al.*, 1977). The syndrome usually occurs within 24 h of commencing total PN following a period of malnutrition. Starting at half the proposed rate of delivery, with slow increments to achieve the nutritional goal, has been suggested to prevent the syndrome. However, recommended levels of monitoring generally ensure that any disturbance is recognized, and the syndrome is now rarely seen.

Complications of lipid infusions

Pulmonary function

Rapid infusion of lipids has been associated with transient but significant declines in arterial oxygen saturation (Patel *et al.*, 1984). The mechanism is uncertain, but may be related to the role of linoleic acid as a precursor of arachidonic acid. Reductions in arterial oxygen saturation have not been observed when lipid is delivered as a gradual infusion over 12 to 24 h.

Hepatic dysfunction related to lipid infusion

Hepatic enzyme abnormalities have occurred when high rates (> 2.5 g/kg/day) of lipid are infused. However, patients with hepatic dysfunction may be unable to deal with much lower levels of lipid, leading to hyperlipidaemia and cholestasis (Allardyce, 1982). Awareness of the problem and high levels of suspicion are essential. The simple test of allowing a blood sample to stand for 20 min and inspecting it for a lipid layer ensures that any problem will be picked up quickly. However, there is rarely a problem if the lipid is infused over 24 h. Fasting triglyceride levels can be measured and if >10%, intralipid should be substituted for 20%.

Reticulo-endothelial function

Infusions of lipid have been associated with impaired reticulo-endothelial function in animals (Hirschberg *et al.*, 1990). This is thought to be related to rates of clearance of long-chain triglycerides from the reticulo-endothelial cells, and gradual accumulation of long-chain triglycerides in the liver. The problem is alleviated if medium-chain triglycerides are substituted. However, evidence in humans is lacking, and overall the effect on immune function is unclear.

Hepatic dysfunction

Parenteral nutrition has been found to cause periportal fatty infiltration and glycogen accumulation. The patient exhibits elevated liver enzyme activity and bilirubin levels. If PN continues, periportal inflammation and portal fibrosis may result after 4–8 weeks, with clinical signs of abdominal pain, hepatomegaly and liver tenderness. These signs are also associated with cholestasis (see below), and should be differentiated from it. The aetiology of these abnormalities is unknown, but could be associated with a dextrose content which is in excess of the patient's capacity for glucose oxidation, thus leading to glycogen and triglyceride synthesis. These substances may sequestrate in the hepatic tissues, producing fatty infiltration. However, there are obviously other factors involved as this does not occur with enteral nutrition. It is also more likely to occur in septic patients, possibly due to carnitine deficiency (Kaminski *et al.*, 1980).

The current provision of non-protein calories in a two-thirds glucose:one-third lipid ratio and the trend towards lower calorie volumes (1500–2500 kcal/day) should reduce the likelihood of hepatic dysfunction.

Cholestasis and acalculous cholecystitis

Patients who have received PN for more than 3 weeks may be at risk of developing cholecystitis.

Clinical symptoms associated with cholecystitis include:

- diffuse or right upper quadrant abdominal tenderness;
- fever;
- leukocytosis;
- high serum bilirubin.

Cholestasis occurs as a result of:

- decreased frequency of gall-bladder contraction caused by diminished jejunal cholecystokinin release due to a lack of enteral stimulus (Doty *et al.*, 1985);
- reduced bile flow associated with PN (Innis, 1985).

Cholestasis and the formation of sludge and/or gallstones are significantly associated with cholecystitis. Both acalculous and calculous cholecystitis can occur, and high levels of awareness are required to ensure early recognition of the problem.

Peripheral parenteral nutrition (PPN)

The administration of central PN is not without problems. Thus the administration of PN via the peripheral route is an attractive alternative, despite the risk of thrombophlebitis and associated complications.

Complications of PPN include:

- peripheral vein thrombophlebitis;
- catheter occlusion;
- venous thrombosis;
- dislodgement;
- sepsis.

Peripheral vein thrombophlebitis

Peripheral vein thrombophlebitis (PVT) is defined as the presence of two or more of the following signs:

- pain;
- swelling;
- erythema;
- excessive warmth;
- palpable venous cord (Khawajia *et al.*, 1991; Payne-James, 1993).

The development of PVT is identified by the presence of inflammation, subsequent thrombosis and occlusion of the peripheral vein, with associated changes in the overlying skin, when a cannula has been placed in a vein. This definition is useful in clinical practice, and provides a focus for the nutrition nurse specialist or clinician. In research-based studies, a quantitative system is used where each sign is measured at different points in relation to the cannula (Table 9.3).

Factors causing PVT include:

- catheter material;
- catheter size;
- vein size;
- insertion technique;
- frequency of change of catheter;
- osmolarity and pH of nutrient solution.

Table 9.3 Maddox criteria (adapted from Maddox *et al.*, 1977)

Score	Criteria
0	No pain at i.v. site, no erythema, no swelling, no induration, no palpable venous cord
1	Painful i.v. site, no erythema, no swelling, no induration, no palpable venous cord
2	Painful i.v. site with erythema, or some degree of swelling, or both, no induration, no palpable venous cord
3	Painful i.v. site with erythema and swelling, and with induration or a palpable venous cord less than 3 inches above i.v. site
4	Painful i.v. site, erythema, swelling, induration and a palpable venous cord more than 3 inches above i.v. site
5	Frank vein thrombosis together with all signs of (4). i.v. infusion may have stopped running due to thrombosis

Interventions which minimize PVT in relation to the above include the following.

1. Use polyurethane rather than silicone and teflon (Kohlhardt *et al.*, 1991; Madan *et al.*, 1992; Everitt *et al.*, 1993).
2. Use a small-gauge cannula/catheter (22 g or 23 g) (Madan *et al.*, 1992; Everitt *et al.*, 1993).
3. Use the largest vein available, e.g. basilic, cephalic median–antecubital fossa (Madan *et al.*, 1992; Colagiovanni, 1996).
4. Use one experienced clinician or nutrition nurse specialist for insertion of the cannula/catheter (Colagiovanni, 1996).
5. Change the cannula/catheter every 12 h (not practical) (Kevin *et al.*, 1991).
6. Use nutrient solutions with minimal osmolarity and a pH of 7.2–7.4 (Messing *et al.*, 1986).

Further interventions which minimize PVT include the use of glyceryl trinitrate (GTN) and lipid emulsions.

It has been suggested that infusion phlebitis is initiated by venoconstriction at the infusion site. Thus the use of a vasodilator may reduce its incidence (Hecher *et al.*, 1984) and prevent platelet aggregation by stimulating prostacyclin (Khawajia *et al.*, 1991). The use of 5-mg GTN patches may not be advisable in patients with renal impairment, glaucoma and/or an unstable cardiovascular system. GTN patches are currently used in the administration of PPN, together with the correct type and size of catheter and low osmolarity of the PPN solution. GTN patches (5–15 mg) are placed near to the vessel and may remain *in situ* for up to 48 h. A minor complication of their use is headache. Analgesics may be sufficient to relieve the headache, but if this is not the case, a reduction in the dose of the GTN patch is both feasible and practical. The addition of lipid emulsion to the glucose solutions buffers the vein wall and reduces endothelial injury (Khawajia *et al.*, 1991).

Catheter occlusion

This is a common problem. To prevent it from occurring, it is important to maintain a continuous flow within the narrow lumen of the catheter. PN bags should always be changed promptly after each infusion. If this is not possible, then heparinized saline (50 units in 5 mL) should be administered before and after infusion.

Catheter-related sepsis

This is defined as a clinical episode of systemic illness with isolation of an identical organism from both catheter tip and peripheral blood in the absence of any obvious primary infective source (Kohlhardt *et al.*, 1991). CRS is rare in the administration of PPN, due to good insertion techniques by an experienced operator and subsequent quality line care.

Dislodgement

Great care must be taken when inserting a peripheral PN cannula. Catheters should either be sutured in position or, more commonly, anchored with steristrips and an occlusive film dressing. Subsequently care should be taken when positioning the patient's forearm in order to prevent dislodgement. There is no need for frequent routine catheter dressings, as frequent dressings have no bearing on the incidence of PVT, and only serve to increase the risk of catheter dislodgement. However, if there is pain, an accumulation of blood or serous fluid, the dressing should be removed with caution and the site inspected.

References

Allardyce, D.B. 1982: Cholestasis caused by lipid emulsion. *Surgery, Gynaecology and Obstetrics* **154**, 641–7.

Armstrong, C.W., Mayhall, C.G. and Muller, K.B. 1986: A prospective study of catheter replacement and other risk factors for infection of hyperalimentation catheters. *Journal of Infectious Diseases* **154**, 808–16.

Berger, R. and Adams, L. 1989: Nutritional support in the critical care setting. Part 2. *Chest* **96**, 372–80.

Colagiovanni, L. 1996: Peripheral benefits. *Nursing Times* **92**, 59–64

Cottee, S. 1995: Heparin lock practice in total parenteral nutrition. *Professional Nurse* **11**, 25–9.

De Ciccio, M., Chiaradia, V., Veronesi, A. *et al.*, 1989: Source and route of microbial colonization of parenteral nutrition catheters. *Lancet* **10**, 1258–61.

Doty, J.E., Pitt, H.A., Porter-Fink, V. *et al.* 1985: Cholecystokinin prophylaxis of parenteral nutrition-induced gall-bladder disease. *Annals of Surgery* **201**, 76–80.

Elliot, T.S.J., Faroqui, M.H., Armstrong, R. and Hanson, G. 1994: Guidelines for good practice in central venous catheterization. *Journal of Hospital Infection* **28**, 163–76.

Everitt, N., Madan, M., Alexander, D.J. and McMahon, M. 1993: Fine bore silicone rubber and polyurethane catheters for the delivery of complete intravenous nutrition via a peripheral vein. *Clinical Nutrition* **12**, 261–5.

Freund, H. and Rimon, B. 1990: Sepsis during total parenteral nutrition. *Journal of Parenteral and Enteral Nutrition* **14**, 39–40.

Grimble, G., Payne-James, J., Rees, R. and Silk, D. 1989: Total parenteral nutrition – clinical applications. *Intensive Therapy and Clinical Monitoring* **January**, 19–26.

Hecher, J.F., Fisk, G.C. and Lewis, G.B.H. 1984: Phlebitis and extravasation ('tissuing') with intravenous infusions. *Medical Journal of Australia* **140**, 658–60.

Hirschberg T., Pomposelli, J.J., Mascioli, E.A., Bistrian B.R. and Blackburn, G.L. 1990: Effect of tracer and intravenous fat emulsion on the measurement of reticulo-endothelial system function. *Journal of Parenteral and Enteral Nutrition* **14**, 463–6.

Innis, S.M. 1985: Hepatic transport of bile salt and bile composition following total parenteral nutrition with and without lipid emulsion in the rat. *American Journal of Clinical Nutrition* **41**, 1283–8.

Ioannides-Demos, L.L., Liolios L., Topliss, D.J. and Mclean, A.J. 1995: A prospective audit of total parenteral nutrition at a major teaching hospital. *Medical Journal of Australia* **163**, 233–7.

Johnson, S. 1994: A time and money saver? Cost comparison of IV therapy with and without IV PALL 96 filters. *Professional Nurse* **10**, 94–6.

Kaminski, D.L., Adams, A. and Jellinek, M. 1980: The effect of hyperalimentation on hepatic lipid content and lipogenic enzyme activity in rats and man. *Surgery* **88**, 93–100.

Kevin, M., Pickford, I., Jaegar, H. *et al.* 1991: A prospective and randomised study comparing the incidence of infusion phlebitis during continuous and cyclic peripheral parenteral nutrition. *Clinical Nutrition* **10**, 315–9.

Khawajia, H., Williams, J. and Weaver, P. 1991: Transdermal glyceryltrinitrate to allow peripheral total parenteral nutrition: a double-blind placebo-controlled feasibility study. *Journal of the Royal Society of Medicine* **84**, 69–72.

Kohlhardt, S.R., Smith, R.C. and Wright, C.R. 1994: Peripheral versus central intravenous nutrition: comparison of two delivery systems. *British Journal of Surgery* **81**, 66–70.

Krzywda, E.A., Andris, D.A., Whipple, J.K. *et al.* 1993: Glucose response to abrupt initiation and discontinuation of total parenteral nutrition. *Journal of Parenteral and Enteral Nutrition* **17**, 64–7.

Lin, M.T., Saito, H., Fukushima, R. *et al.*, 1996: Route of nutritional supply influences local, systemic and remote organ responses to intraperitoneal bacterial challenge. *Annals of Surgery* **223**, 84–93.

Linares, J., Sitges-Serra, A., Garau, J., Perez, J.L. and Martin, R. 1985: Pathogenesis of catheter sepsis. A prospective study with quantitative and semi-quantitative cultures of catheter hub and segments. *Journal of Clinical Microbiology* **21**, 357–60.

Madan, M., Alexander, D.J. and McMahon, M. 1992: Influence of catheter type on occurrence of thrombophlebitis during peripheral intravenous nutrition. *Lancet* **339**, 101–3

Maddox, R., Rush, D., Rapp, K. *et al.* 1977: Double-blind study to investigate methods to prevent cephalothin-induced phlebitis. *American Journal of Hospital Pharmacy* **34**, 29–34.

Maki, D.G. and Will, L. 1984: Colonization and infection associated with transparent dressings for central venous, arterial and Hickman catheters: a comparative trial. Proceedings of 24th

Interscience Conference on Antimicrobial Agents and Chemotherapy, American Society for Microbiology.

Maki, D.G., Wheeler, S. and Stolz, S. 1990: Prospective study of a novel, transparent highly permeable polyurethane dressing for intravascular catheters. Proceedings of the Hospital Infection Society Meetings

Messing, B., Leveve, M., Rigaud, D. *et al.* 1986: Peripheral venous complications of a hyperosmolar nutritive mixture: the effect of heparin and hydrocortisone. A multicentre double-blind random study in 98 patients. *Clinical Nutrition* **5**, 57–61.

Murphy, L. and Lipman, T. 1987: Central venous catheter care in parenteral nutrition – a review. *Journal of Parenteral and Enteral Nutrition* **11**, 190–201.

Norwood, S., Allan R., Civetta J. and Cortes V. 1991: Catheter-related infections and associated septicaemia. *Chest* **99**, 968–75.

Patel, C.B, Mathru, M. and Sandoval, E.D. 1984: Pulmonary effects of lipid infusion in patients with acute respiratory failure. *Critical Care Medicine* **12**, 293–5.

Payne-James, J.J. 1993: Peripheral parenteral nutrition: what peripheral vein thrombophlebitis PVT prophylaxis to use? In *Intensive care Britain Vol. 2*. London: Greycoat Publishing, 12–22.

Pennington, C.R. 1996: *Current perspectives on parenteral nutrition in adults*. Biddenden: British Association of Parenteral and Enteral Nutrition.

Pomposelli, J.J. and Bistrian, B.R. 1994: Is total parenteral nutrition immunosuppressive? *New Horizons* **2**, 224–9.

Powell, C., Regan, C., Fabin, P. and Roberg, R. 1982: Evaluation of opsite catheter dressings for parenteral nutrition: a prospective, randomized trial. *Journal of Parenteral and Enteral Nutrition* **6**, 43–6.

Roberts, P.H. 1993: Simply a case of good practice: avoiding catheter-related sepsis in total parenteral nutrition. *Professional Nurse* **8**, 775–9.

Sitges-Serra, A., Linares, J. and Garav, J. 1984a: Catheter sepsis: the clue is the hub. *Surgery* **97**, 355–7.

Sitges-Serra, A., Puig, P., Linares, J. *et al.* 1984b: Hub colonization as the initial step in an outbreak of catheter-related spesis due to coagulase negative staphylococci during parenteral nutrition. *Journal of Parenteral and Enteral Nutrition* **8**, 668–72.

Sitzman, J.V., Townsend, T.R., Siler, M.C. and Bartlett, J.G. 1985: Septic and technical complications of central venous catheterization: a prospective study of 200 consecutive patients. *Annals of Surgery* **202**, 766–70.

Stotter, A., Ward, H., Natesfield, A., Hilton, J. and Sim, A. 1987: Junctional care: the key to prevention of catheter sepsis in intravenous feeding. *Journal of Parenteral and Enteral Nutrition* **11**, 159–62.

Torosian, M.H., Meranze, S., McClean, G. and Mollen, J.L. 1986: Central venous access with occlusive superior central vein thrombosis. *Annals of Surgery* **203**, 30–3.

Tovey, S.J. Benton, K.G.F. and Lee, H.A. 1977: Hypophosphataemia and phosphorus requirements during intravenous nutrition. *Postgraduate Medical Journal* **53**, 287–9.

Wolfe, B.M., Ryder, M.A., Nishikawa, R.A., Halsted, C.H. and Schmidt, B.F. 1986: Complications of parenteral nutrition. *American Journal of Surgery* **152**, 93–9.

Nutritional rehabilitation

The aims of this chapter are:

- to outline the steps to returning to oral nutrition;
- to identify the problems associated with regaining dietary health following critical illness;
- to highlight the problems faced by patients once they move from the ICU.

Introduction

'Rehabilitation embraces the many physical, social and organisational aspects of the aftercare of most patients who require more than acute, short-term definitive care' (Nicols, 1980).

'Rehabilitation means the restoration of the individual to the fullest mental, social, vocational and economic capacity of which he is capable' (National Council on Rehabilitation - USA).

'Rehabilitation is the restoration of patients to their fullest physical, mental and social capability' (Mair, 1992).

These definitions highlight the physical, social, physiological and economic components of an individual's life. Therefore, it is sensible that in order for rehabilitation to be effective, it must begin as early as possible. This allows both the patient and the carer, together with the appropriate health care professionals working within nutrition to be sympathetic to the future needs of the patient.

However, this early rehabilitation programme is often difficult to achieve in the initial days of a patient's admission to the intensive-care unit, because of the multifaceted problems associated with critical illness and the need for support modalities.

In the critically ill patient, normal metabolism is interrupted by periods of catabolism which may be compounded by poor levels of nutritional intake. Within a short period of time, the sequence of events resulting from the catabolic and hypermetabolic response leads to severe muscle wasting and a loss of body stores. Strategies to prevent catabolism and aid recovery have already been reviewed (see chapter 2).

Thus notwithstanding the treatment and care given to a patient for his or her initial diagnosis, other problems will naturally occur. These are associated with the profound reduction in nutrient stores and supply associated with a period of critical illness.

The most significant effects of this reduction are:

- weight loss;
- skeletal muscle wasting;
- disturbed respiratory and cardiac muscle function;
- immunosuppression;
- increased risk of nosocomial infection;
- delay in wound healing and repair (Griffiths, 1992).

Although the loss of contractile protein delays weaning from mechanical ventilation in the short term, the longer-term consequences are also important. The resultant reduced activity and prolonged bed rest can ultimately lead to a prolonged convalescence and a delay in the patient regaining his or her independence and a return to a normal daily life (Griffiths, 1992).

Many studies have been undertaken in the past, recording data on morbidity and mortality, long-term outcomes and quality of life in the intensive-care setting (Sage *et al.*, 1986; Dragsted, 1990). However, there is little information available on the recovery period in the weeks following discharge (Benzer *et al.*, 1983; Daffurn *et al.*, 1994), and even less on outcome measures assessing the efficacy of nutritional supplementation of critically ill patients.

The transition from critical care to the general ward

It is important to stress that during the critical-care episode there is a strong emphasis on supportive rather than repletional nutrition. A clear understanding of what has gone before, in terms of nutritional repletion and illness, is necessary to determine the pace of nutritional rehabilitation. This is perhaps best set up with the early involvement of the hospital nutrition team and/or the nutrition nurse specialist, starting in the ICU.

The team can supply advice on nutritional delivery, cannulae, dressings and steps to progression back to an oral diet. In addition, they can give psychosocial support to the patient and provide patient and carer training if there is a need to continue nutritional support after discharge. The nutrition team will also monitor and review the patient's nutritional status and ensure that complications are either avoided or quickly recognized.

Problems that need to be overcome include the following:

- physical disability, i.e. lack of appetite, dysphagia associated with tracheal intubation and possible stricture, reduction in gastric volume;
- lack of control over food intake and desire to eat;
- regaining the social perception of eating.

The patient will need to work his or her way back to perceiving nutritional intake as a part of social interaction. The steps are as follows.

1. Food is provided (artificial nutritional support) and is outside the patient's control.
2. Food is eaten in order to survive and perhaps at the urging of others. There is minimal patient control.
3. Food is enjoyed and the patient makes active choices regarding the food eaten.
4. Food becomes a social occasion, and the patient interacts with others around a meal.

Promoting nutritional rehabilitation in ICU

Griffiths (1992) undertook a study to investigate how nutritional intervention can be assessed. The findings of this study were as follows.

1. This type of assessment depended on strong criteria, a well-defined protocol, a randomized selection process for patients, and exclusion criteria which were realistic and applicable.
2. Outcome measures were difficult to define. Short-term indices of successful nutritional treatment included a reduction in muscle

wasting, improved gastrointestinal function, and a reduction in the incidence of infection.
3. Patients and community health care professionals seemed more interested in the effectiveness of treatment in terms of survival and the quality of life experienced than in terms of nutritional outcome.

This apathy towards nutrition may in part explain why there is a difficulty in continuing data collection on outcome. This is because the nutritional needs of the critically ill patient once achieved in intensive care can be neglected when the patient has been transferred to a general ward.

The transition from ICU to the general ward

Problems to overcome include:

- premature discontinuation of nutritional support;
- lack of or poor monitoring of oral nutritional intake;
- intolerance of an oral diet following artificial nutrition support;
- partial or intermittent dysphagia due to prolonged intubation and insertion of a tracheostomy.

In this latter situation, early speech therapy intervention is required to improve swallowing and increase confidence in eating, in most cases normally following a dependence on artificial feeding.

Action plan

1. Record intake daily on specific oral nutrition charts.
2. Continue with artificial nutrition support until oral intake is up to at least 50 per cent of target requirements.
3. Consider overnight nasogastric feeding to supplement oral intake.
4. Ensure that the dietitian and nutritional support team are aware of the patient both on the ICU and following transfer to the ward.
5. Review target requirements as patient mobility improves. Increased activity requires increased intake.

Post discharge from hospital

Both Griffiths (1992) and Daffurn *et al.* (1994) have highlighted the need for follow-up intensive-care clinics which provide continual assessment, diagnosis, treatment, counselling and support for patients whose admission to intensive care was for longer than 5 days.

Problems experienced by patients following ICU admission have been identified as belonging to two categories.

Physical problems

These include:

- sensory neuropathy;
- fine motor control disturbance;
- visual and hearing disturbance;
- loss of appetite;
- loss of taste;
- skin and hair disorders;
- sexual dysfunction.

Psychological problems

These include:

- anxiety;
- depression;
- hallucinations;
- sleep disturbance;
- confusion;
- social isolation;
- irritability.

Jones *et al.* (1994) recorded that patients in the ICU follow-up clinics, when asked, could not remember anything about their stay in intensive care. She thus concluded that the most important time for psychological support is not while patients are in intensive care, but once they are discharged home, as it has been suggested that the discharge home is the most psychologically stressful phase of critical illness. This is due to the high levels of social isolation and irritability, coupled with a possible loss of income, which can have devastating effects on a family. It is therefore important that on discharge from the ICU/HDU, the patient continues to be monitored and supported by experienced health care professionals, whether this is at home or on the general ward.

High levels of support should be gradually reduced in order to allow time, a key element in rehabilitation, for the patient to adapt from the dependent atmosphere of the intensive-care unit to individually controlling his or her own health and destiny.

NUTRITION AND DIETETIC SERVICE
PATIENT FOOD RECORD CHART

Patient Name ...John Bellow............ Ward ...Bonco - Jonpa.............

Date ....

| The patient is having (Please tick) | Small portions ☐ | High protein soup ☐ |
| | High protein pudding ☐ | Diabetic pudding ☐ |

DAY AFTER ADMISSION

	Description (quantity)	1/4	1/2	3/4	All	kcal	Protein
Breakfast							
Cereals, milk, sugar (tsp)	1 bowl cornflakes, milk				✓		
Eggs							
Bread (slices)	1 slice				✓		
Butter, margarine, jam	Butter x 1, Jam x 1				✓		
Tea, coffee, milk, sugar (tsp), fruit juice	Tea with milk				✓		
Other (e.g. supplements) Maxijul, Ensure, Build-up, etc.							
Mid-morning							
Tea, coffee, milk, sugar (tsp)	Tea with milk				✓		
Biscuits							
Other (e.g. supplements) Maxijul, Ensure, Build-up, etc.							
Lunch							
Soup	Vegetable, 1 bowl				✓		
Cheese, egg, meat, fish, pulses	Lancashire hot pot			✓			
Vegetables	carrots				✓		
Potatoes, rice, pasta, bread	portion boiled potato				✓		
Dessert, fruit	Jelly x 1				✓		
Drinks	Tea with milk				✓		
Other (e.g. supplements) Maxijul, Ensure, Build-up, etc.							
Mid-afternoon							
Tea, coffee, milk, sugar (tsp)	Tea with milk				✓		
Biscuits							
Other (e.g. supplements) Maxijul, Ensure, Build-up, etc.							
Supper							
Soup	Tomato, 1 bowl				✓		
Cheese, egg, meat, fish, pulses							
Vegetables							
Potatoes, rice, pasta, bread							
Dessert, fruit							
Drinks							
Sandwiches	Chicken salad x 1				✓		
Other (e.g. supplements) Maxijul, Ensure, Build-up, etc.							
Bedtime							
Milky drink, sugar (tsp)	Hot chocolate x 1				✓		
Tea, coffee, milk, sugar (tsp)							
Biscuits							
Other (e.g. supplements) Maxijul, Ensure, Build-up, etc.							

Fig. 10.1 Nutrition and Dietetic Service Patient Food Record chart.

Case study

Mr Bellow has been transferred from the ICU to the ward. His requirements have recently been reviewed and are now 2500 kcal/ day.

Figure 10.1 is a record of his intake.

Calculate the number of kcalories he has consumed and compare this with his requirement. If the requirement is not met, calculate the quantity of supplements he will need to meet his nutritional goal.

References

Benzer, H., Mutz, N. and Pauser, N. 1983: Psychosocial sequelae in intensive care. *International Anaesthetic Clinics* **21**, 169–78.

Daffurn, K., Bishop, G., Hillman, K.M. and Bauman, A. 1994: Problems following discharge after intensive care. *Intensive and Critical Care Nursing* **10**, 244–51.

Dragsted, L. 1990: Long-term outcome from intensive care. In Vincent, J.L. (ed.) *Update in intensive care emergency medicine Vol. 10.* Berlin: Springer, 865–9.

Griffiths, R.D. 1992: Development of normal indices of recovery from critical illness. In Rennie, M. (ed.) *Intensive care Britain.* London: Greycoat Publishing, 134–7.

Jones, C., Griffiths, R. Macmillan, R. and Palmer, T. 1994: Psychological problems occurring after intensive care. *British Journal of Intensive Care* **4**, 46–50.

Sage, W.M., Rosenthal, M.H. and Silverman, J.F. 1986: Is intensive care worth it? An assessment of input and outcome for the critically ill. *Critical Care Medicine* **14**, 777–82.

Further reading

Lavery, G., Scott, A., Shaffer, J. *et al.* 1993: Consensus workshop on enteral feeding of ICU patients. *British Journal of Intensive Care* **3**, 438–47.

Nichols, P.J.R. 1980: *Rehabilitation medicine: the management of physical disabilities.* 2nd edn. London: Butterworth.

Striker, R. 1997: *Rehabilitation aspects of acute and chronic nursing care.* 2nd edn. Philadelphia: WB Saunders.

Index

NOTE: this index is arranged alphabetically word by word. Page numbers in *italics* refer to tables or diagrams.